PEDIATRICS, CHILD AND ADOLESCENT HEALTH

CHINESE ADOLESCENT DEVELOPMENT

ECONOMIC DISADVANTAGES, PARENTS AND INTRAPERSONAL DEVELOPMENT

PEDIATRICS, CHILD AND ADOLESCENT HEALTH

JOAV MERRICK –SERIES EDITOR –

NATIONAL INSTITUTE OF CHILD HEALTH AND HUMAN DEVELOPMENT, MINISTRY OF SOCIAL AFFAIRS, JERUSALEM, ISRAEL

Child and Adolescent Health Yearbook 2012
Joav Merrick (Editor)
2012. ISBN: 978-1-61942-788-4

Child Health and Human Development Yearbook 2011
Joav Merrick (Editor)
2012. ISBN: 978-1-61942-969-7

Tropical Pediatrics: A Public Health Concern of International Proportions
Richard R Roach, Donald E Greydanus, Dilip R Patel, Douglas N Homnick and Joav Merrick (Editors)
2012. ISBN: 8-1-61942-831-7

Developmental Issues in Chinese Adolescents
Daniel TL Shek, Rachel CF Sun and Joav Merrick (Editors)
2012. ISBN: 978-1-62081-262-4

Positive Youth Development: Theory, Research and Application
Daniel TL Shek, Rachel CF Sun and Joav Merrick (Editors)
2012. ISBN: 978-1-62081-305-8

Understanding Autism Spectrum Disorder: Current Research Aspects
Ditza A Zachor and Joav Merrick (Editors)
2012. ISBN: 978-1-62081-353-9

Positive Youth Development: A New School Curriculum to Tackle Adolescent Developmental Issues
Hing Keung Ma, Daniel TL Shek and Joav Merrick (Editors)
2012. ISBN: 978-1-62081-384-3

Transition from Pediatric to Adult Medical Care
David Wood, John G Reiss, Maria E Ferris, Linda R Edwards and Joav Merrick (Editors)
2012. ISBN: 978-1-62081-409-3

Child and Adolescent Health Yearbook 2011
Joav Merrick (Editor)
2013. ISBN: 8-1-61942-782-2

Child Health and Human Development Yearbook 2012
Joav Merrick (Editors)
2013. ISBN: 978-1-61942-978-9

Chinese Adolescent Development: Economic Disadvantages, Parents and Intrapersonal Development
Daniel TL Shek, Rachel CF Sun and Joav Merrick (Editors)
2013. ISBN: 978-1-62618-622-4

University and College Students: Health and Development Issues for the Leaders of Tomorrow
Daniel TL Shek, Rachel CF Sun and Joav Merrick (Editors)
2013. ISBN: 978-1-62618-586-9

Adolescence and Behavior Issues in a Chinese Context
Daniel TL Shek, Rachel CF Sun and Joav Merrick (Editors)
2013. ISBN: 978-1-62618-614-9

Advances in Preterm Infant Research
Jing Sun, Nicholas Buys and Joav Merrick (Editors)
2013. ISBN: 978-1-62618-696-5

Promotion of Holistic Development of Young People in Hong Kong
Daniel TL. Shek, Tak Yan Lee and Joav Merrick
2013. 978-1-62808-019-3

Internet Addiction: A Public Health Concern in Adolescence
Artemis Tsitsika, Mari Janikian, Donald E Greydanus, Hatim A Omar and Joav Merrick (Editors)
2013. ISBN: 978-1-62618-925-6

Human Developmental Research: Experience from Research in Hong Kong
Daniel TL Shek, Cecilia Ma, Yu Lu and Joav Merrick (Editors)
2013. ISBN: 978-1-62808-166-4

Chinese Adolescent Development: Economic Disadvantages, Parents and Intrapersonal Development
Daniel TL Shek, Rachel CF Sun and Joav Merrick (Editors)
2013. ISBN: 978-1-62618-622-4

PEDIATRICS, CHILD AND ADOLESCENT HEALTH

CHINESE ADOLESCENT DEVELOPMENT

ECONOMIC DISADVANTAGES, PARENTS AND INTRAPERSONAL DEVELOPMENT

DANIEL T. L. SHEK
RACHEL C. F. SUN
AND
JOAV MERRICK
EDITORS

nova publishers
New York

For permission to use material from this book please contact us:
Telephone 631-231-7269; Fax 631-231-8175
Web Site: http://www.novapublishers.com

Library of Congress Cataloging-in-Publication Data

Chinese adolescent development : economic disadvantages, parents and intrapersonal development / editors, Daniel T.L. Shek, Rachel C.F. Sun and Joav Merrick (Health Services, Division for Intellectual and Developmental Disabilities, Ministry of Social Affairs and Social Services, Jerusalem, Israel, and others).
pages cm
Includes index.
ISBN 978-1-62618-622-4 (hardcover)
1. Teenagers--China--Social conditions. 2. Adolescence--China. 3. Youth development--China. 4. Adolescent psychology--China. I. Shek, Daniel T. L. II. Sun, Rachel C. F. III. Merrick, Joav, 1950-
HQ799.C55C515 2013
305.2350951--dc23

2013013150

Published by Nova Science Publishers, Inc. † New York

Contents

INTRODUCTION
NEGLECTED RESEARCH ON CHINESE ADOLESCENT DEVELOPMENT

For adolescents in the contemporary world, poverty and economic problems are not new events to them. Since the Asian financial crisis which took place in 1997, several other global financial problems occurred in the past 15 years. These included the 2000 Internet bubble, 2008 Wall Street bubble in the United States, and the European debt crisis in 2011. With globalization and fluctuations in the financial markets, unemployment and job instability are growing concerns faced by many countries. Unfortunately, despite the growing problem of poverty in many countries and the negative consequences of poverty on adolescent development, the study of poverty "has not been accorded the level of research attention as families in middle class" (1, p. 589). Luthar (2) also remarked "there is a need for greater attention to theoretical conceptualizations regarding 'normative development' in the context of poverty" (p. 579).

With specific reference to the Chinese culture, Shek (3,4) pointed out that with a few exceptions (5,6), there is a paucity of research studies on adolescents experiencing economic disadvantage. One example is that when the search term "poverty" was used, computer search in January 2012 using PsycINFO showed that there were 8,948 citations. However, when the search terms "poverty" and "Chinese" were used, there were only 88 citations (i.e. about 1% of the total related citations). As Chinese people constitute roughly one-fifth of the world's population, the proportion of Chinese research in this area is on the low side.

There are several areas of research that should be conducted with reference to Chinese adolescents experiencing economic disadvantage. First, there is a need to understand how factors in different ecological systems influence the psychological well-being of poor adolescents. Second, as family social capital is an important resource within families experiencing economic disadvantage, studies on how different family processes affect adolescent development should be carried out. In particular, as parental sacrifice and motivation to study are strongly emphasized in the Chinese culture, related studies with reference to these issues should be examined. Third, as far as adolescent developmental outcomes are concerned, it is argued that besides measures of morbidity and symptoms, adolescent developmental assets and strengths should be studied. Fourth, as studies on parental differences on family processes are almost non-existent in the context of poverty, it is important to study this issue in adolescents experiencing economic disadvantage. In response to these research gaps, they were examined in the papers in this special issue.

Another neglected area of research concerns holistic development among university students. A survey of the literature shows that there are many developmental issues in university students (7,8). Based on the notion of universal prevention in the public health approach, it is argued that development and implementation of subjects focusing on psychosocial competencies and holistic development is a promising approach. Unfortunately, although there are many validated positive youth development programs for high school students (9-13), there are comparatively fewer related programs for university students. Hence, it is important to ask how we can develop more related programs for university students.

At The Hong Kong Polytechnic University, a new subject entitled "Tomorrow's Leaders" has been designed to promote holistic development in students admitted under the New Undergraduate Curriculum in 2012/13 academic year. The subject focuses on those positive youth development constructs which are intrinsic to the existing positive youth development programs, particularly the Project P.A.T.H.S. in Hong Kong. Some of these constructs include emotional competence, cognitive competence, resilience, spirituality, positive identity and interpersonal communication.

To get some implementation experience of the subject and to evaluate its effectiveness, the subject was piloted in 2010/11 academic year, with four classes of students taking this subject. Several evaluation strategies, including objective outcome evaluation, post-course subjective outcome evaluation, post-lecture subjective outcome evaluation, process evaluation, qualitative evaluation using reflective notes and focus group evaluation were employed. Overall speaking, the evaluation findings were very positive which clearly suggest that the subject was able to promote holistic development in the students taking this subject (14-19).

To consolidate the subject and to further examine its effectiveness, the subject was piloted for the second time in the first term of 2011/12 academic year. Again, several evaluation strategies were adopted. First, a quasi-experimental design with an experimental group and a control group was used. Second, post-course subjective outcome evaluation was conducted. Third, post-lecture subjective outcome evaluation data were collected. Fourth, qualitative evaluation based on reflective notes was conducted. Fifth, qualitative evaluation based on personal reflections was adopted. Sixth, focus groups were conducted to examine the experiences of the students. Finally, process evaluation via systematic observations was carried out.

This book is based upon a special issue published in the International Journal on Disability and Human Development (21) and permission has been obtained from the publisher De Gruyter in Berlin to publish this modified version of the papers in this book.

In this book, several papers reporting evaluation findings for the second piloting exercise are included. Because there are few validated positive youth development programs in the Chinese context (20), it is our modest wish that the accumulated evidence can give us some insights about the usefulness of having positive youth development subjects designed for university students.

Chair Professor Daniel TL Shek, PhD, FHKPS, BBS, JP
Department of Applied Social Sciences, The Hong Kong Polytechnic University, Hunghom, Hong Kong, P.R.China E-mail: daniel.shek@polyu.edu.hk

Assistant Professor Rachel CF Sun, PhD
Faculty of Education, The University of Hong Kong, Pokfulam Road, Hong Kong, P.R.China E-mail: rachels@hku.hk

Professor Joav Merrick, MD, MMedSci, DMSc
National Institute of Child Health and Human Development, Division for Intellectual and Developmental Disabilities, Ministry of Social Affairs and Social Services, Jerusalem, Israel.
E-mail: jmerrick@zahav.net.il

REFERENCES

[1] Orthner, DK. Families in poverty: key issues for research. J Fam Issues 1996;17:588-92.

[2] Luthar SS. Sociodemographic disadvantage and psychological adjustment: perspectives from developmental psychopathology. In: Luthar SS, Burack JA, Cicchetti D, editors. Developmental Psychopathology. New York: Cambridge University Press 1997:459-585.

[3] Shek DTL. Paternal and maternal influences on the psychological well-being, substance abuse, and delinquency of Chinese adolescents experiencing economic disadvantage. J Clin Psychol 2005;61:219-34.

[4] Shek DTL. Quality of life research: responses to emerging issues in a changing world. Soc Indic Res 2011;100:371-4.

[5] Shek DTL. Economic stress, psychological well-being and problem behavior in Chinese adolescents with economic disadvantage. J Youth Adolesc 2003;32:259-66.

[6] Shek DTL. Economic stress, emotional quality of life, and problem behavior in Chinese adolescents with and without economic disadvantage. Soc Indic Res 2005;71:363-83.

[7] Shek DTL. Nurturing holistic development of university students in Hong Kong ScientificWorld Journal 2010;10:563-75.

[8] Shek DTL, Wong KK. Do adolescent developmental issues disappear overnight? reflections about holistic development in university students. ScientificWorld Journal 2011;11:353-61.

[9] Shek DTL, Ma CMS, Tang CYP. Predictors of subjective outcome evaluation findings in a positive youth development program in Hong Kong. Int J Disabil Hum Dev 2011;10:249-55.

[10] Shek DTL, Sun RCF, Merrick J. Training programs and implementation process of positive youth development programs. Int J Adolesc Med Health 2011;23:303-4.

[11] Shek DTL, Ma HK, Sun RCF. A brief overview of adolescent developmental problems in Hong Kong. ScientificWorld Journal 2011;11:2243-56.

[12] Shek DTL, Ma HK, Sun RCF. Development of a new curriculum in a positive youth development program: the Project P.A.T.H.S. in Hong Kong. ScientificWorld Journal 2011;11:2207-18.

[13] Sun RCF, Shek DTL. Positive youth development, life satisfaction and problem behaviour among Chinese adolescents in Hong Kong: a replication. Soc Indic Res 2012;105:541-59.

[14] Shek DTL, Sun RCF. Promoting psychosocial competencies in university students: evaluation based on a one group pretest-posttest design. Int J Disabil Hum Dev, in press.

[15] Shek DTL, Sun RCF. Promoting leadership and intrapersonal competence in university students: what can we learn from Hong Kong? Int J Disabil Hum Dev, in press.

Shek DTL, Sun RCF. Process evaluation of a positive youth development course in a university setting in Hong Kong. Int J Disabil Hum Dev, in press.

[16] Shek DTL, Sun RCF. Qualitative evaluation of a positive youth development course in a university setting in Hong Kong. Int J Disabil Hum Dev, in press.

[17] Shek DTL, Sun RCF. Focus group evaluation of a positive youth development course in a university in Hong Kong. Int J Disabil Hum Dev, in press.

[18] Shek DTL. Post-lecture evaluation of a positive youth development subject for university students in Hong Kong. ScientificWorld Journal, in press.
[19] Shek DTL, Yu L. Prevention of adolescent problem behavior: longitudinal impact of the Project P.A.T.H.S. in Hong Kong. ScientificWorld Journal 2011;11:546-67.
[20] Shek DTL, Sun RCF, Merrick J. Quality of life of Chinese adolescent5s: Missing research gaps. Int J Disabil Hum Dev 2013;12(2).

Economic Disadvantage and Hong Kong

In: Chinese Adolescent Development ISBN: 978-1-62618-622-4
Editors: Daniel TL Shek, Rachel CF Sun, Joav Merrick © 2013 Nova Science Publishers, Inc.

Chapter 1

ARE FAMILY PROCESSES RELATED TO ACHIEVEMENT MOTIVATION OF CHINESE ADOLESCENTS EXPERIENCING ECONOMIC DISADVANTAGE IN HONG KONG?

Janet TY Leung, BSSc, MA, PhD, RSW[1]
and Daniel TL Shek, PhD, FHKPS, BBS, JP[*] [1,2,3,4,5]
[1]Department of Applied Social Sciences,
The Hong Kong Polytechnic University, Hong Kong, PRC
[2]Centre for Innovative Programmes for Adolescents and Families,
The Hong Kong Polytechnic University, Hong Kong, PRC
[3]Kiang Wu Nursing College of Macau, Macau, PRC
[4]Department of Social Work, East China Normal University,
Shanghai, PRC
[5]Division of Adolescent Medicine,
Kentucky Children's Hospital, University of Kentucky,
Lexington, United States of America

ABSTRACT

The relationships between perceived parenting style, parental control, family functioning, parental sacrifice for children's education and achievement motivation were examined in 275 Chinese adolescents experiencing economic disadvantage in Hong Kong. Consistent with the hypotheses, parenting style, parental control, family functioning, and parental sacrifice for children's education were related to adolescent achievement motivation. Regression analyses further showed that maternal control, as well as paternal and maternal sacrifice for children's education were significant predictors of achievement

[*] Correspondence: Professor Daniel TL Shek, PhD, FHKPS, BBS, JP, Chair Professor of Applied Social Sciences, Faculty of Health and Social Sciences, Department of Applied Social Sciences, The Hong Kong Polytechnic University, Room HJ407, Core H, Hunghom, Hong Kong. E-mail: daniel.shek@polyu.edu.hk.

motivation of adolescents experiencing economic disadvantage. Theoretical and practical implications of the findings are discussed.

INTRODUCTION

Poverty has been a social concern in the global context. There are many theoretical accounts postulating that poverty impairs family processes which further adversely affect adolescent development (1-3). According to Atkinson's theory (4) on motivation, motivation consists of two components: the desirability of an outcome and the expectancy that one can attain it. In the path of poverty, people perceive themselves as facing uncontrollable circumstances. According to Kane (3), learned helplessness perceived by individuals experiencing poverty involves "motivational deficit" (believing action is useless), "cognitive interference" (difficulty in learning that action can produce positive outcomes in new situations) and "affective reaction" (depression or resignation). Pareek (5) further elaborated the model by suggesting that poverty induced a specific pattern of motivation with low need for achievement, low need for extension and high need for dependence. This motivational pattern together with expectancy of powerlessness created the lifestyle and culture of poverty. The outcomes included disproportionate risk taking, interest in chance, lack of interest in feedback, seeking of peers with similar frustrations, lack of activity and initiative, lack of regard for others, lack of faith and trust, avoidance behaviors, fear of failure, seeking favors of superiors and over-conformity. Interestingly, this analysis echoes the Chinese belief of "*ren qong zhi duan*" (poverty stifles ambition), which clearly portraits the harmful effect of poverty on one's motivation.

Facing the harmful impacts of poverty on individual's motivation, one may raise the following questions: While economically disadvantaged children and adolescents face the problems in motivation, why do some perform so well? Where does their driving force come from? What enables them to escape from the influences of poverty and strive for achievement? Actually, these questions have been raised by researchers and theorists in the field of resilience. Research based on the "positive development" perspective does not necessarily focus on the negative impacts of poverty on adolescent development. Garmezy (6) suggested three categories of protective factors that moderated the influence of poverty on adolescent developmental outcomes. These include: (1) personality/dispositional features, such as self-esteem, locus of control, self-efficacy, optimum, active coping strategies; (2) affectional ties within the families, such as cohesion, warmth, shared values, patience, consistency of rules, and support from adults; and (3) availability of external support systems such as schools, churches and caring agencies. Echoing these suggestions, other researchers also indicated that familial qualities and processes are important in buffering the impacts of poverty on the development of economically disadvantaged adolescents (7-10).

A review of the literature showed that there are several limitations pertinent to the research on the relationships between family processes and adolescent's motivation in economically disadvantaged families. First, there is a severe lack of studies examining achievement motivation in adolescents experiencing economic disadvantage. To understand adolescent's motivation to perform, achievement motivation is one of the important developmental attributes that contribute to the positive development of adolescents; it is especially important for economic disadvantaged adolescents because achievement motivation is a "hope-oriented" attribute (11) that steers adolescents to succeed. Unfortunately, research on achievement motivation of Western and Chinese adolescents in the context of poverty is almost non-existent. It is of fundamental importance to understand familial protective factors that predict achievement motivation of adolescents experiencing economic disadvantage because this may give cues for combating intergenerational poverty.

Besides, another problem concerning achievement motivation is its conceptualization. Most research employed Western conceptualization of achievement motivation that favors an "individualistic orientation" in determining achievement goals, incentive value of success, standard of excellence and criteria of evaluation. Unfortunately, many scholars criticized that the "individualistic" concept of achievement motivation was unsuitable for Chinese people, which are rooted in collectivist orientation of Confucian philosophy (12,13). Hence, the conceptualization and measurement of achievement motivation should reflect a Chinese cultural orientation that emphasizes on externally determined goals or standards of excellence that are socially defined and approved (13).

Similarly, many Chinese researchers employed Western concepts of family processes in their studies. Shek (14) queried about the compatibility of Western theories and research findings when applied to Chinese people because Western family concepts and theories built on individualistic values that may not be compatible with the collectivistic ideology of Chinese families. Chao (15) also criticized Western descriptions of Chinese parenting for being "rather ethnocentric and misleading" (p. 1111). Yang (16) argued that the unquestioning borrowing of Western concepts and tools results in the inhibition of native values, views and ways of thinking. Hence, there is an urgent need to develop indigenous Chinese conception of family processes and parenting. For example, Chao and Tseng (17) identified three central themes for Asian parenting: centrality of the family and family interdependence, parental control and strictness, and fostering of educational achievement of children.

Methodologically speaking, the problems of conceptualization of achievement motivation and family processes bring forth the problems of measurement tools. There is a severe lack of psychosocial assessment tools in the Chinese culture (18,19). Indigenous measurement tools that accurately capture Chinese conceptions of achievement motivation and family processes are also rare in the literature.

The final limitation of the related research is that the impact of family processes on adolescent development is a complex process that involves more than one pathway (20). Furthermore, it is unclear which family process is comparatively more important in promoting adolescent achievement motivation than other processes. To address this issue, Shek (21) suggested that we should examine different aspects of parenting because they "can reveal the complex nature of the linkage between parenting and adolescent psychological well-being" (p. 273).

How may family processes affect adolescent achievement motivation? The expectancy-value theory on motivation and socialization model of children's motivation and achievement suggested by Eccles et al. (22,23) may give us insight into the mechanisms and development of motivation. The expectancy-value theory on motivation assumes that motivation is directly determined by the relative value and probability of success of various options (expectancies). The expectancies and values are influenced by ones' beliefs such as perceptions of competence, perceptions of task difficulty, individual's goals and self schemas. These social cognitive variables are in turn influenced by other peoples' expectations and behaviors (22).

With reference to socialization of children's motivation and achievement, parents influence the expected outcomes of their children via their parenting strategies. There are four components of parenting that are worth highlighting: 1) developmentally appropriate timing of achievement demands/pressure, 2) high confidence in children's abilities, 3) a supportive affective family climate, and 4) highly motivated role models (22, p. 1052). The first and second components are related to the expectations, standards, and demands of parents for their children. These contribute to parenting styles and practices. The third component is related to parenting qualities and home environment for socialization. The fourth component is concerned about parents' role modeling. There are empirical research findings that parenting styles and practices (24-27), warm and stable family environment with affectional family relationships (28,29), and parental involvement (30-32) predicted motivation and educational achievement of adolescents.

With specific reference to the Chinese culture, it is noteworthy that parental control and parental sacrifice are distinctive features of Chinese parenting (17,33). There are studies showing that parental control fostered educational achievement of children and adolescents in Chinese societies (24,34), though research on economically disadvantaged families were minimal. Moreover, qualitative studies also discovered parental sacrifice for child's education influenced motivation and educational achievement of adolescents (35-37). Unfortunately, quantitative Chinese studies on understanding the relationships of parental sacrifice and achievement motivation of Chinese adolescents are also non-existent. Thus, it is interesting and illuminating to study the relationships of different family processes including parenting style, parental control, parental sacrifice for children's education, and family functioning with adolescent achievement motivation in Chinese economically disadvantaged families.

In this study, two research questions were formulated. The first question is: are there any relationships between family processes and achievement motivation of economically disadvantaged adolescents? Based on socialization model and the expectancy-value theory on motivation (22,23) as well as previous research findings, seven hypotheses were formulated in this study. It was hypothesized that: a) more positive perceived paternal and maternal endorsement of parenting styles would be related to higher achievement motivation of adolescents (Hypothesis 1a and 1b); b) higher levels of perceived paternal and maternal control would be associated with higher achievement motivation of adolescents (Hypothesis 1c and 1d); c) more perceived paternal and maternal sacrifice for children's education would be associated with higher achievement motivation of adolescents (Hypothesis 1e and 1f); and d) a higher level of family functioning would be associated with higher achievement motivation of adolescents (Hypothesis 1g).

The second research question is: what is the relative importance of family processes in predicting achievement motivation of Chinese adolescents experiencing economic disadvantage? As research on this area is non-existent, it is theoretically and practically interesting to explore the relative importance of dyadic family processes and systemic family functioning in predicting adolescent achievement motivation.

OUR STUDY

A cross-sectional survey with purposeful sampling was conducted. Adolescents aged 11 to 16 from intact families experiencing economic disadvantage were invited to participate in the study. The concept of relative poverty was adopted, with 50% of monthly median domestic household income according to the Hong Kong Population By-census 2006 was used as the poverty threshold. The economic disadvantaged families were identified and recruited by children and youth service centers, school social work services, and community centers across Hong Kong. Finally, 276 families participated in the study. There was one adolescent questionnaire that was found to be invalid, thus 275 adolescent questionnaires were analyzed.

Either the first author or trained social workers conducted the data collection. Adolescents were given explanations about the purpose of the research, procedure of data collection, the rights of respondents to voluntarily participate and withdraw from the study, as well as the use of the data in the study. Informed consent from both parents and adolescents was obtained. Adolescents were requested to complete the Adolescent Questionnaires which contained measures of parenting styles, parental control, family functioning, parental sacrifice for children's education and achievement motivation. The questionnaire was administered in a self-administered format. Adolescents took around 35 minutes to complete the questionnaires.

There were 134 boys (48.7%) and 141 girls (51.3%) who participated in the study. The ratio was close to that of secondary schools (51.3: 48.7) in Hong Kong according to the 2006 Population By-census. The mean age of the adolescents was 13.56 (*SD* = 1.54), with the mean of boys and girls at 13.40 (*SD* = 1.60) and 13.71 (*SD* = 1.47) respectively. There were 18 adolescents (6.5%) studying in Primary Five or below (Grade 5 and below), 47 (17.1%) in Primary Six (Grade 6), 63 (22.9%) in Secondary One (Grade 7), 46 (16.7%) in Secondary Two (Grade 8), 42 (15.3%) in Secondary Three (Grade 9), 28 (10.2%) in Secondary Four (Grade 10), and 29 (10.5%) in Secondary Five and above (Grade 11 and above). Regarding the duration of stay in Hong Kong, 144 adolescents (52.4%) were born in Hong Kong, and 74 (27.0%) had resided in Hong Kong for more than 7 years. But still, 24 (8.7%) adolescents had resided in Hong Kong for less than 3 years.

As for the family profile, the mean ages of the fathers and mothers were 49.94 (*SD* = 9.28) and 42.18 (*SD* = 4.97), respectively. Most fathers were born in Hong Kong (n = 98, 35.6%) or had resided in Hong Kong for more than 20 years (n = 115, 41.8%), whereas the mode of duration of stay of mothers in Hong Kong was between 6 and 10 years (n = 103, 37.5%). Regarding the educational attainment of fathers and mothers, a majority were of low educational standard, with 205 fathers (74.5%) and 204 mothers (74.2%) at the junior secondary level or lower. There were 211 (76.7%) fathers who had a job, 30 (10.9%) were unemployed, and 26 (9.5%) had retired. A high proportion of mothers were housewives (n = 199, 72.4%). The average number of children in the families was 2.34 (*SD* = .90). There were 96 families receiving Comprehensive Social Security Assistance from the Government, occupying 34.8% of the sample.

Instruments

Paternal Parenting Style Scale (APPS) and Maternal Parenting Style Scale (AMPS). Base on the framework of Maccoby and Martin (38) and parenting assessment work of Lamborn et al. (39), Shek (40) developed a modified version of the Paternal/Maternal Parenting Style Scale (APPS/AMPS). There are two subscales of this scale, including Paternal/Maternal Demandingness Scale (PDEM/MDEM) which assesses the demandingness of the father and mother towards the child's behaviors, and Paternal/Maternal Responsiveness Scale (PRES/MRES) which assesses the responsiveness of the father and mother to the child's behaviors. There are 7 items in the Demandingness Scale and 13 items in the Responsiveness Scale. The scales were found to be valid and reliable in the Chinese culture (40,41). Higher Paternal/Maternal Parenting Style Scale scores indicate more positive parental attributes. Reliability analyses showed that both APPS and AMPS had satisfactory reliability in this study ($\alpha = 0.856$ and 0.834, respectively).

Chinese Paternal Control Scale (APCS) and Chinese Maternal Control Scale (AMCS). Based on a review of the literature, Shek (42,43) developed a twelve-item Chinese Paternal/Maternal Control Scale to assess control based on indigenous Chinese cultural concepts. Adolescents were requested to rate the degree of agreement with each item on a 4-point scale ranging from "Strongly agree" to "Strongly disagree". Examples of the items are "My father expects me to be mature (*sheng xing*)"; "My father expects me to have good behavior so that I will not bring dishonor to the family (*you ru jia sheng*)". The APCS and AMCS showed internal consistency and divergent validity (43). The total score of the items in each scale is an indicator of the degree of parental control based on Chinese concepts, with a higher score indicating a higher level of Chinese parental control. Reliability analyses showed that both APCS and AMCS had satisfactory reliability in this study ($\alpha = .870$ and .876, respectively).

Paternal/Maternal Sacrifice for Children's Education Scale (APSA/AMSA). Based on the literature on family investment (44), family capital (45,46), and parental involvement in children's education (47,48), as well as qualitative findings from focus groups of parents and adolescents respectively, an indigenous scale assessing parental sacrifice for children's education was developed (49). The scale was developed with 23 items measuring dimensions of sacrifice in terms of financial resources, time on children's education, reorganization of daily routine, sacrifice of lifestyle and aspiration, and shielding from worries. Participants were requested to rate the degree of agreement with each item on a 6-point Likert scale ranging from "Strongly agree" to "Strongly disagree". Examples of the items are "To fulfill my educational needs, my father eats and wears less"; "Even if my father is tired, he tries his/her best to understand my school life". Both APSA and AMSA showed internal consistency, divergent validity and factorial validity in a previous validation study (50). Higher scores indicate greater parental sacrifice for children's education. Reliability analyses showed that both APSA and AMSA had high reliability in this study ($\alpha = .938$ and .942, respectively).

The Chinese Family Assessment Instrument (AFAI). The AFAI is an indigenous 33-items self-report instrument assessing family functioning in Chinese populations. The C-FAI has five subscales – mutuality, communication, conflict and harmony, parental concern, and parental control. Higher scores indicate higher levels of family functioning. Shek and his colleagues (51,52) performed a series of validation studies that examined the factor structure, reliability, concurrent, and discriminant validity of C-FAI and showed that that the scale was a valid and reliable measure of family functioning in the Chinese community. The scale was demonstrated to have excellent reliability in this study ($\alpha = .949$).

Social Oriented Achievement Motivation (SOAM) Scale. Social Oriented Achievement Motivation (SOAM) scale is a self-reported culture-specific measure of Chinese achievement tendencies developed by Yu and Yang (13). The SOAM scale contains 30 items that measures four aspects of achievement motivation: achievement value, achievement goal, achievement related behaviors and outcome evaluation. The SOAM scale emphasizes goals and evaluation criteria defined by significant others, groups, and society (53). Examples of SOAM scale items are “In order not to disappoint my parents, I always try to do what they expect” and “The main goal of my life is to do things that will make my parents feel proud”. Responses to the item statements are reported on a 6-point Likert scale where 1= totally disagree and 6= totally agree. The scale has good internal consistency, test-retest reliability, convergent validity and discriminant validity (13). The total score of the items in the scale is an indicator of the degree of social-oriented achievement motivation, with higher scores indicating higher levels. The scale was demonstrated to have good reliability in this study ($\alpha = .944$).

FINDINGS

To analyse the relationships between family processes and adolescent achievement motivation, Pearson correlation analyses were performed. In order to decrease the chance of committing Type I error, a conservative alpha level based on Bonferroni correction (alpha = .05/7, i.e. .007) was adopted. When assessing the correlations of demographic data with adolescents’ perception of family processes and achievement motivation, it was found that perceived paternal parenting style (APPS) were significantly associated with age of adolescents ($r = -.275$, $p < .001$) and educational level of adolescents ($r = -.224$, $p < .001$), suggesting that older, more educated adolescents had lower endorsement of perceived positive paternal parenting styles. The amount of overlap on the correlation of APPS on age and educational level of adolescents were 7.56%, and 5.02% of the variance, respectively. Thus, partial correlations of APPS scores by age of adolescents and educational levels of adolescents were computed. Similarly, perceived maternal parenting style (AMPS) was significantly associated with age of adolescents ($r = -.303$, $p < .001$) and educational level of adolescents ($r = -.246$, $p < .001$), suggesting that older, more educated adolescents had lower endorsement of positive maternal parenting style. The amount of overlap on the correlation of AMPS and age and educational level of adolescents were 9.18%, and 6.05% of the variance, respectively. Therefore, partial correlations of AMPS scores by age of adolescents and educational level of adolescents were computed. Moreover, adolescents’ perception of family functioning (AFAI) was significantly related to their status of receiving CSSA ($r = -.216$, $p < .001$), suggesting that those families receiving CSSA would have relatively lower family functioning perceived by adolescents. The amount of overlap on the correlation of AFAI and status of CSSA recipient was 4.67% of the variance. Hence, partial correlation of AFAI scores by status of CSSA recipient was suggested.

Research Question 1

Results showed that perceived positive endorsement of paternal and maternal parenting styles were associated significantly with achievement motivation of economically disadvantaged adolescents, with Pearson's *r* at .253 ($p < .001$) and .259 ($p < .001$) respectively. The relationships remained significant when age and educational level of adolescents were controlled. Hence, Hypotheses 1a and 1b were supported.

Perceived paternal and maternal control were also correlated with achievement motivation of adolescents, with Pearson's *r* at .308 ($p < .001$) and .393 ($p < .001$). The effect size was between medium to great. Hypotheses 1c and 1d were supported.

Perceived paternal and maternal sacrifice for children's education were associated significantly with achievement motivation of economically disadvantaged adolescents, with Pearson's *r* of .402 ($p < .001$) and .425 ($p < .001$) respectively. The effect sizes were between medium to large. Hypotheses 1e and 1f were supported.

Finally, it was found that family functioning was associated significantly with their achievement motivation, with Pearson's *r* of .220 ($p < .001$). With the control of status of CSSA recipients, the value of Pearson's *r* reduced to .203 ($p < .007$), which still indicated significant correlation.

Table 1 shows the correlations between the family processes and achievement motivation of adolescents experiencing economic disadvantage.

Table 1. Correlations between relative family processes and achievement motivation perceived by adolescents experiencing economic disadvantage

		Adolescents						
		Perceived parental parenting style		Perceived parental control		Perceived family functioning	Perceived parental sacrifice for children's education	
		APPS	AMPS	APCS	AMCS	AFAI	APSA	AMSA
Adolescents	SOAM	.253*** (.222***)[a]	.259*** (.225***)[a]	.308***	.393***	.220*** (.203**)[b]	.425***	.367***

Note 1. *** $p < .001$.

Note 2. [a] The number in parentheses was the correlation coefficient calculated after age and educational level of adolescents were controlled. [b] The number in parentheses was the correlation coefficient calculated after status of CSSA recipients was controlled.

Note 3. APPS= Perceived Paternal Parenting Style Scale. AMPS= Perceived Maternal Parenting Style Scale. APCS= Perceived Paternal Control Scale. AMCS= Perceived Maternal Control Scale. APSA= Perceived Paternal Sacrifice for Children's Education Scale. AMSA= Perceived Maternal Sacrifice for Children's Education Scale. AFAI= Perceived Family Assessment Inventory. SOAM= Social Oriented Achievement Motivation Scale.

Research Question 2

Hierarchical regression analyses were performed to understand the relative importance of different family processes on achievement motivation of adolescents experiencing economic disadvantage. Demographic variables (age and educational levels of adolescents, status of

CSSA recipients), family processes (paternal and maternal parenting styles, paternal and maternal control, paternal and maternal sacrifice for children's education, and family functioning) were entered into hierarchical blocks. It was found that perceived maternal control ($\beta = .265$, $p < .001$), paternal and maternal sacrifice for children's education ($\beta = .262$, $p < .01$ and $\beta = .162$, $p < .05$, respectively) were significant predictors of achievement motivation of adolescents. Table 2 shows the results of hierarchical regression analyses of adolescent achievement motivation in economically disadvantaged families. Figure 1 lists the prediction of different family processes on the achievement motivation of adolescents.

Table 2. Hierarchical regression analyses of achievement motivation of adolescents experiencing economic disadvantage

	Step 1 (β)	Step 2 (β)
Age of adolescents	-.024	.025
Educational level of adolescents	-.153	-.093
CSSA status	-.110	-.086
Paternal parenting style		-.042
Maternal parenting style		.056
Paternal control		-.022
Maternal control		.265***
Paternal sacrifice for children's education		.262**
Maternal sacrifice for children's education		.162*
Family functioning		-.038
F	4.047	10.704
R^2	.043	.288
ΔR^2		.246

β = Standardized regression coefficient.
*$p < .05$, ** $p < .01$, *** $p < .001$.

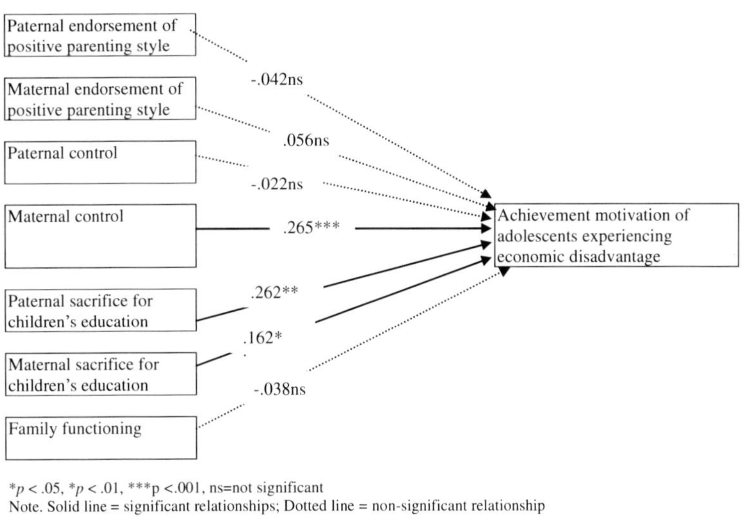

*$p < .05$, *$p < .01$, ***p <.001, ns=not significant.
Note. Solid line = significant relationship; Dotted line = non-significant relationship.

Figure 1. Predictions of different family processes on achievement motivation of adolescents experiencing economic disadvantage.

Discussion

The present findings support the socialization models of motivation (22) that family processes predict achievement motivation of adolescents. As proposed by Eccles et al. (22), developmentally appropriate achievement demands, as well as a supportive affective family climate, are important components in the socialization of motivation of adolescents. Thus, positive endorsement of parenting style with parental responsiveness and demandingness, parental control of children's behaviors, and better family functioning were essential in predicting adolescent achievement motivation. Furthermore, parental investment and involvement were also essential in enhancing the achievement motivation of adolescents, though these result in parental sacrifice of parents' personal needs. It was found that the influences of family processes (paternal and maternal parenting style, paternal and maternal control, paternal and maternal sacrifice for children's education, and family functioning) were substantial in building achievement motivation of economically disadvantaged adolescents.

Among different family processes perceived by adolescents, it was found that paternal and maternal sacrifice for children's education and maternal control showed the greatest association with achievement motivation of adolescents. Qualitative studies on parental sacrifice give us some insight on the explanation on how parental sacrifice enhances achievement motivation of economically disadvantaged adolescents. In her qualitative study on how higher education students broke through the intergenerational cycle of education level inheritance, Gofen (36) found that children felt indebted to their parents' sacrifice and thus regarded it a duty to fulfil the parents' expectations. Fuligni and Yoshikawa (35) also found that a sense of filial obligation motivated children and adolescents to achieve academically and avoid problem behaviors in response to the sacrifice of parents who had migrated to the United States for a better future. The studies indicated that children who were deeply indebted to parents' sacrifice would be motivated to achieve out of gratitude to their parents' unconditional love. This view echoes the "reciprocity" concept of fulfilling different roles within the Chinese family system, as indicated by mutual care and obligation (17). Parents hold the authority and responsibility for taking care of their children, and children in turn are obliged to respect their parents and fulfil their responsibility to the families. It should be noted that paternal sacrifice for children's education had greater effect size on association with adolescents' achievement motivation than did maternal sacrifice. As adolescents perceived that their fathers made a lot of sacrifices to engage in unpleasant jobs and long hours of work with their low educational and socio-economic background in order to earn a living, they were more motivated for achievement and more motivated to strive for a better future so that they could eventually support the family and to honour their fathers for their sacrifice and investment. Thus, adolescents may be more indebted to the fathers' devotion and sacrifice and are thus motivated towards achievement in return. In view of the fact that related studies are almost non-existent in the global context, it is important to conduct more research in this area.

Another significant predictor of adolescent achievement motivation was maternal control of children's behaviors. To account for the influence of maternal control in influencing achievement motivation of adolescents, the concepts of filial piety and shame strategy may give us some insight. As mentioned, parental control is distinctive in Chinese parenting practices for setting parental expectation and standards in monitoring children's behaviors

(15,17). Adolescents are expected to follow the standards and expectations of parents in the pursuit of filial piety. Moreover, "shame" strategy was an indigenous Chinese socialization practice (54,55). When parents execute clear expectations and standards for adolescents, those who fail would experience shame and guilt. Thus, adolescents may put effort into achievement in order to gain pride and reduce shame to their families. Obviously, this is also a manifestation of filial piety (53). As mothers spent more time and effort nurturing their children than fathers, adolescents would be more sensitive to the expectations and standards of mothers. In manifesting filial piety as well as avoiding shame that would disgrace the families and create disappointment for their mothers, adolescents were motivated to achieve for the sake of the families. In addition, it was found that the emphasis of interdependence in the Chinese family system was more salient in mother-child relationships, as Chinese mothers emphasized the relational goals of fostering enduring mother-child relationships and sharing of love and affection (17). Thus, adolescents were more sensitive to mother-child relationships and experienced more shame and guilt for failing to fulfil their mothers' instructions and standards. With the fear of hurting their mothers and breaking the mother-child relationships, adolescents were motivated to strive for achievement.

It is noteworthy that there are different roles of fathers and mothers in enhancing the achievement motivation of economically disadvantaged adolescents. Fathers, as breadwinners, are responsible for protecting family members and striving for family resources for maintenance of family daily necessities and adolescent development. Thus, paternal sacrifice for children's education is an important family process that enhances achievement motivation of adolescents. This is particularly important for poor families, as fathers put extraordinary effort into striving for financial resources for family expenses and their children's development. The process may involve extra paternal sacrifice, as resources for poor families are scarce. Mothers, on the other hand, are mainly responsible for child-rearing roles such as caring, nurturing and monitoring children's behaviors in the families. As the child-rearing role is central to mothers' responsibilities, maternal control is considered a significant predictor of achievement motivation of adolescents. The findings echo with the cultural inclination of "*nan zhu wai, nu zhu nei*" (men manage things outside the family, whereas women manage things inside the families) in Chinese community. The differential contributions of fathers and mothers to adolescent achievement motivation via paternal sacrifice and maternal control are illuminating for us to understand the complex family processes of poor families.

There are several theoretical and practical implications of the study. First, as studies on adolescent achievement motivation in economic disadvantage families are almost non-existent, the present study is a pioneering contribution to the literature. Second, the study underscores the importance on using indigenous concepts that fit the unique Chinese context. The concepts of achievement motivation, parental control, family functioning and parental sacrifice for children's education are indigenous and unique in the Chinese context where collectivistic orientation and Confucian thought is stressed. The findings suggest that maternal control and parental sacrifice for children's education, which are the distinctive features of Chinese parenting practices (17,33), are the most influential family processes that enhance achievement motivation of adolescents experiencing economic disadvantage. The study demonstrates the importance of employing indigenous Chinese concepts in building Chinese family models.

Third, this study suggests that different family processes in relation to adolescent achievement motivation should be studied in the context of poverty. To conceptualize the complexity of family processes and family relationships, dyadic (father-adolescent, mother-adolescent) family processes including parenting style, parental control, parental sacrifice for children's education, as well as systemic family processes of family functioning should be explored. While the family processes provide us important information on the contributions and different roles of fathers and mothers in parenting their children, the family relationships address the interdependence among family relationships. As only few studies in the literature included both dyadic and systemic family processes in a single study (56,57), the present study is the first scientific study that explored both dyadic and systemic processes of economically disadvantaged families in the Chinese community.

Fourth, as a large majority of poverty research employed the "deficiency" paradigm and focused on the detrimental effects of poverty to the families and adolescents (58-62), the protective factors of family processes on adolescent development in economically disadvantaged families were usually ignored. The present study highlights the importance of focusing on achievement motivation of Chinese adolescents experiencing economic disadvantage, which is an important attribute of positive development of adolescents. The study identified the family processes that were critical factors in enhancing achievement motivation of economically disadvantaged adolescents, which gives us new light on helping adolescents to beat the odds of poverty, and resolving the problems of intergenerational poverty.

Fifth, the findings provide important cues on family intervention in helping economically disadvantaged families. Instead of taking a residual model on providing tangible support for the families, or putting emphasis solely on adolescents in overcoming the odds of poverty, the research findings suggest that parents do "make a difference" on enhancing achievement motivation of adolescents experiencing economic disadvantage. Thus, the findings suggest the importance of adopting a family-based intervention approach to help the economically disadvantaged families. Family-life education, emotional and instrumental support for parents and parenting enhancement programs would be necessary for parents to build up achievement motivation of adolescents.

Sixth, it was found that paternal parenting style, paternal control, and paternal sacrifice were significantly associated with achievement motivation of adolescents. The findings suggest that the roles and involvement of fathers should be strengthened. However, long hours of work, low educational standard and cultural inclinations hinder fathers' involvement in parenting. To help adolescents and families living in poverty, participation of fathers in parenting is essential. Social workers have to reach out to engage fathers in family education programs. Men service should be expanded to cover parenting and roles of families.

Last but not least, the different roles of fathers and mothers on enhancing adolescent achievement motivation imply a call for gender-sensitive practice in family intervention for economically disadvantaged families. The different roles of fathers and mothers entail different needs of fathers and mothers. Fathers, responsible for mobilizing family resources for the families, may experience great pressure as their wages are minimal. They may perceive themselves and be perceived by others as incompetent and inadequate in their family roles. On the other side, mothers take up more parental roles on monitoring and control, in addition to the conventional expectations of caring and nurturing. As "higher behavioral control would be physically and psychologically taxing for mothers" (63, p. 679), mothers may shoulder most burden in monitoring and nurturing their children. The strains and stresses of performing family roles may affect the psychological well-being of fathers and mothers, and may cause marital conflict. Social workers and clinical practitioners should be sensitive to the different roles of fathers and mothers and address their psychological and parenting needs.

Although this is the first known scientific study examining the relationships between family processes and achievement motivation in adolescents experiencing economic disadvantage, there are several limitations of the present study. First, the limitation of purposeful sampling should be realized. As adolescents were not randomly sampled, generalizability of the findings may be limited. Second, the cross-sectional design in this study has the inherent problem in inferring cause-and-effect relationships due to the lack of time order. Hence, a longitudinal research design is recommended in future studies. Third, as the assessment of family processes was based on self-reported measures, the findings may only represent the perceptions of the "insiders". Thus, it would be more illuminating to include the observation data in real-life settings from the "outsiders" view so that a more comprehensive picture of linkage between family processes and adolescent achievement motivation in Chinese families experiencing economic disadvantage can be obtained. Fourth, the information collected was based on adolescents only. Day, Gavazzi, and Acock (64) argued that considering responses from just one person in family research provides "a very limited basis for extrapolating a sequence of events that may lead to a certain decision or interactional style" (p. 110). Information based on multiple informants such as parents would be desirable. Last but not least, as the findings presented in the study were based on economically disadvantaged adolescents in Hong Kong, there is a need to assess the generalizability of the findings in different Chinese communities (e.g. mainland China) and Chinese people living in non-Chinese contexts (e.g. Chinese-Americans).

Despite these limitations, the present findings are pioneering and stimulating in view of the paucity of research in studying the relationships between family processes and achievement motivation of Chinese adolescents experiencing economic disadvantage. Essentially, the study is an active and constructive response that provides some clues on enhancing adolescent achievement motivation and preventing adolescents from falling into the tragedy that "poverty trifles ambition". The present findings clearly show that besides strengthening the psychosocial competencies of adolescents themselves which would eventually promote the developmental outcomes of adolescents (65-69), helping parents is an important intervention point for promoting the adjustment of adolescents experiencing economic disadvantage.

ACKNOWLEDGMENTS

This chapter has been published as a paper in the International Journal on Disability and Human Development, 2013;12(2). Permission has been obtained from De Gruyter to re-publish in this modified form.

References

[1] Conger RD, Conger KJ. Understanding the processes through which economic hardship influences families and children. In: Crane DR, Heaton TB, eds. Handbook of families and poverty. Los Angeles: Sage, 2008:64-81.

[2] Duncan GJ, Raudenbush SW. Assessing the effects of context in studies of children and youth development. Educ Psychol 1999;34:29-41.

[3] Kane TJ. Giving back control: Long-term poverty and motivation. Soc Serv Rev 1987;63(3):405-19.

[4] Atkinson JW. An introduction to motivation. Princeton, NJ: Nostrand, 1964.

[5] Pareek U. Poverty and motivation: Figure and ground. In: Dalal AK, Misra G, eds. New directions in Indian psychology: Social psychology, Vol. 1. New Dalhi: Sage, 2002:262-79.

[6] Garmezy N. Children in poverty: Resilience despite risk. Psychiatry 1993;56:127-36.

[7] Masten AS, Best KM, Garmezy N. Resilience and development: Contributions from the study of children who overcome adversity. Dev Psychopathol 1990;2:425-44.

[8] Rutter M. Psychosocial resilience and protective mechanisms. Br J Psychiatry 1987;147:589-611.

[9] Rutter M. Psychosocial resilience and protective mechanisms. In: Rolf J, Masten AS, Cicchetti D, Nuechterlein KH, Weintraub S, eds. Risk and protective factors in the development of psychopathology. UK: Cambridge Univ Press, 1990:181-214.

[10] Werner EE, Smith RS. Overcoming the odds: High risk children from birth to adulthood. Ithaca, NY: Cornell Univ Press, 1992.

[11] Feather NT. The relationship of expectation of success to need achievement and test anxiety. J Pers Soc Psychol 1965;1:118-216.

[12] de Vos GA. Socialization for achievement: Essays on the cultural psychology of the Japanese. Berkeley: Univ Calif Press, 1973.

[13] Yu AB, Yang KS. Social-oriented and individual-oriented achievement motivation: conceptualization and measurement. Paper presented at the symposium on Chinese personality and social psychology. 24th International Congress of Psychology, Sydney, 1988.

[14] Shek DTL. Chinese family research: Puzzles, progress, paradigms, and policy implications. J Fam Issues 2006;27(3):275-84.

[15] Chao RK. Beyond parental control and authoritarian parenting style: Understanding Chinese parenting through the cultural notion of training. Child Dev 1994;65:1111-9.

[16] Yang KS. Towards an indigenous Chinese psychology: A selective review of methodological, theoretical, and empirical accomplishments. Chinese J Psychol 1999;41(2):181-211.

[17] Chao RK, Tseng V. Parenting in Asians. In: Bornstein MH, ed. Handbook of parenting. Vol. 4: Social conditions and applied parenting, Mahwah, NJ: Lawrence Erlbaum Associates Publishers, 2002:59-93.

[18] Shek DTL. Quality of life of Chinese people in a changing world. Soc Indic Res 2010;95:357-61.

[19] Shek DTL, Lam MC, Tsoi KW. Evidence-based practice in Hong Kong. In: Thyer B, Kazi MAF, eds. International perspectives on evidence-based practice in social work London: Venture Press, 2004:167-81.

[20] Bradley RH, Corwyn RF. Socioeconomic status and child development. Annu Rev Psychol 2002;53:371-99.

[21] Shek DTL. Paternal and maternal influences on the psychological well-being of Chinese adolescents. Genet Soc Gen Psychol Monogr 1999;125(3):269-96.

[22] Eccles JS, Wigfield A, Schiefele U. Motivation to succeed. In: Damon W, Eisenberg N, eds. Handbook of child psychology, Vol. 3: Social, emotional and personality development, 5th ed. New York: John Wiley, 1998:1017-97.

[23] Eccles JS, Poeser R, Vida M, Fredricks J, Wigfiled A. Motivational and achievement pathways through middle childhood. In: Balter L, Tamis-Lemonda CS, eds. Child psychology: A handbook of contemporary issues. New York: Taylor Francis, 2006:325-55.

[24] Chao RK, Sue S. Chinese parental influence and their children's school success: A paradox in the literature on parenting styles. In: Lau S, ed. Growing up the Chinese way --- Chinese child and adolescent development. Hong Kong: The Chinese Univ Press, 1996:93-120.

[25] Spera C. A review of the relationship among parenting practices, parenting styles, and adolescent school achievement. Educ Psychol Rev 2005;17(2):125-46.
[26] Steinberg L, Elmen JD, Mounts NS. Authoritative parenting, psychosocial maturity, and academic success among adolescents. Child Dev 1989;60:1425-36.
[27] Steinberg L, Lamborn S, Dornbusch S, Darling N. Impact of parenting practices on adolescent achievement: Authoritative parenting, school involvement, and encouragement to succeed. Child Dev1992;63:1266-81.
[28] Furstenberg FF Jr., Cook TD, Eccles J, Elder GH, Jr., Sameroff A. Managing to make it: Urban families and adolescent success. Chicago: Univ Chicago Press, 1999.
[29] Smokowski PR, Reynolds AJ, Bezuckzo N. Resilience and protective factors in adolescence: An autobiographical perspective from disadvantaged youth. J Sch Psychol 1990;37:425-48.
[30] Cooper CE, Crosnoe R. The engagement in schooling of economically disadvantaged parents and children. Youth Soc 2007;38(3):372-91.
[31] Davis-Kean PE. The influence of parent education and family income on child achievement: The indirect role of parental expectations and the home environment. J Fam Psychol 2005;19:698-710.
[32] Englund MM, Egeland B, Collin WA. Exceptions to high school dropout prediction in a low-income sample: do adults make a difference? J Soc Issues 2008;64(1):77-93.
[33] Chao RK, Kaeochinda KF. Parental sacrifice and acceptance as distinct dimensions of parental support among Chinese and Filipino American adolescents. In: Russell ST, Crockett LJ, Chao RK, eds. Asian American parenting and parent–adolescent relationships, New York: Springer Sci Business Media, 2010:61-77.
[34] Cheung CS, McBride-Chang C. Relations of perceived maternal parenting style, practices, and learning motivation to academic competence in Chinese children. Merrill Palmer Quart 2008;54(1):1-22.
[35] Fuligni AJ, Yoshikawa H. Socioeconomic resources, parenting, poverty, and child development among immigrant families. In Bornstein MH, Bradley RH, eds. Socioeconomic status, parenting, and child development. Mahwah, NJ: Lawrence Erlbaum, 2003:107-124.
[36] Gofen A. Family capital: How first-generation higher education students break the intergenerational cycle. Fam Relat 2009;58:104-20.
[37] Weiling E. Do returns on investment for educating children in Oaxaca de Juárez, Mexico, pay off? A qualitative analysis. Int J Qual Stud Educ 2003;16(6):817-34.
[38] Maccoby EE, Martin JA. Socialization in the context of the family: Parent-child interaction. In: Mussen PH, series ed., Hetherington EM, vol. ed. Handbook of child psychology, Vol. 4: Socialization, personality, and social development. New York: Wiley, 1983:1-100.
[39] Lamborn SD, Mounts NS, Steinberg L, Dornbusch SM. Patterns of competence and adjustment among adolescents from authoritative, authoritarian, indulgent, and neglectful families. Child Dev 1991;62:1049-65.
[40] Shek DTL. Parenting characteristics and adolescent psychological well-being: A longitudinal study in a Chinese context. Genet Soc Gen Psychol Monogr 1999;125:27-44.
[41] Shek DTL. A longitudinal study of parenting and psychosocial adjustment among Chinese adolescents experiencing economic disadvantage. Int J Adolesc Med Health 2003;15:39-49.
[42] Shek DTL. Perceived parental control processes, parent-child relational qualities, and psychological well-being in Chinese adolescents with and without economic disadvantages. J Genet Psychol 2005;166(2):171-88.
[43] Shek DTL. Perceived parental control based on indigenous Chinese parental concepts in adolescents in Hong Kong. Am J Fam Ther 2007;35:123-37.
[44] Conger RD, Donnellan MB. An interactionist perspective on the socioeconomic context of human development. Annu Rev Psychol 2007;58:175-99.
[45] Coleman JS. Social capital in the creation of human capital. Am J Sociol 1988;94 (Suppl 95):S95-S120.
[46] Coleman JS. Foundations of social theory. Cambridge, MA: Harvard Univ Press, 1990.
[47] Epstein JL. School and family partnerships. In: Aiken M, ed. Encyclopedia of educational research. New York: Macmillan, 1992:1139-51.

[48] Grolnick W, Benjet C, Kurowski C, Apostoleris N. Predictors of parent involvement in children's schooling. J Educ Psychol 1997;89(3):538-48.
[49] Leung, JTY, Shek DTL. "All I can do for my child" --- Development of the Chinese Parental Sacrifice for Child's Education Scale. Int J Disabil Hum Dev 2011;10(3): 201-08.
[50] Leung, JTY, Shek DTL. Validation of the Chinese Parental Sacrifice for Child's Education Scale. Int J Disabil Hum Dev 2011;10(3):209-15.
[51] Shek DTL. Assessment of family functioning Chinese adolescents: The Chinese Family Assessment Instrument. In: Singh NN, Ollen-dick T, Singh AN, eds. International perspectives on child and adolescent Mental Health. Amsterdam, Netherlands: Elsevier, 2002:297-316.
[52] Siu AMH, Shek DTL. Psychometric properties of the Chinese Family Assessment Instrument in Chinese adolescents in Hong Kong. Adolescence 2005;40:817-30.
[53] Yu AB. Ultimate life concerns, self, and Chinese achievement motivation. In Bond MH, ed. The handbook of Chinese psychology. Hong Kong: Oxford Univ Press, 1996:227-46.
[54] Yang KS. The formation and change of Chinese personality: A cultural-ecological perspective. Acta Psychol Taiwanica 1981; 23:39-55.[Chinese]
[55] Yang KS. Chinese personality and its change. In: Bond MH, ed. The psychology of Chinese people. Hong Kong: Oxford Univ Press, 1986:106-70.
[56] Gjerde PF. The interpersonal structure of family interaction settings: Parent-adolescent relations in dyads and triads. Dev Psychol 1986;22(3):297-304.
[57] Smetana JG, Abernethy A, Harris A. Adolescent-parent interactions in middle-class African American Families: Longitudinal change and contextual variations. J Fam Psychol 2000;14(3):458-74.
[58] Conger RD, Conger KJ, Elder GH Jr., Lorenz FO, Simons RL, Whitbeck LB. A family process model of economic hardship and adjustment of early adolescent boys. Child Dev 1992;63:526-41.
[59] Conger RD, Conger KJ, Elder GH Jr., Lorenz FO, Simons RL, Whitbeck LB. Family economic stress and adjustment of early adolescent girls. Dev Psychol 1993;29(2): 206-19.
[60] Sampson RJ, Laub JH. Urban poverty and the family context of delinquency: A new look at structure and process in a classic study. Child Dev 1994;65:523-40.
[61] Shek DTL. Family life quality and emotional quality of life in Chinese adolescents with and without economic disadvantage. Soc Indic Res 2007;80:393-410.
[62] Shek, DTL. Economic disadvantage, perceived family life quality and emotional well-being in Chinese adolescents: A longitudinal studies. Soc Indic Res 2008;85:169-89.
[63] Shek DTL. Perceived parental control and parent-child relational qualities in early adolescents in Hong Kong: Parent gender, child gender and grade differences. Sex Roles 2008;58:666-81.
[64] Day RD, Gavazzi S, Acock A. Compelling family processes. In: Thornton A. ed. The well-being of children and families – research and data needs. Michigan: Univ Michigan, 2001:103-26.
[65] Shek DTL, Merrick J, eds. Special issue: Positive youth development and training. Int J Adolesc Med Health 2010;21:341-447.
[66] Shek DTL. Subjective outcome and objective outcome evaluation findings: Insights from a Chinese context. Res Soc Work Pract 2010;20:293-301.
[67] Shek DTL, Ma CMS. Impact of the Project P.A.T.H.S. in the junior secondary school years: Individual growth curve analyses. Sci World J 2011;10:253-66.
[68] Shek DTL, Yu L. Prevention of adolescent problem behavior: Longitudinal impact of the Project P.A.T.H.S. in Hong Kong. Sci World J 2011;11:546-67.
[69] Shek DTL, Ng CSM. Early identification of adolescents with greater psychosocial needs: an evaluation of the Project P.A.T.H.S. in Hong Kong. Int J Disabil Hum Dev 2010;9:291-299.

In: Chinese Adolescent Development ISBN: 978-1-62618-622-4
Editors: Daniel TL Shek, Rachel CF Sun, Joav Merrick © 2013 Nova Science Publishers, Inc.

Chapter 2

PARENTING FOR RESILIENCE: FAMILY PROCESSES AND PSYCHOSOCIAL COMPETENCE OF CHINESE ADOLESCENTS EXPERIENCING ECONOMIC DISADVANTAGE IN HONG KONG

***Janet TY Leung, BSSc, MA, PhD, RSW*[1]**
***and Daniel TL Shek, PhD, FHKPS, BBS, JP** [1,2,3,4,5]**
[1]Department of Applied Social Sciences,
The Hong Kong Polytechnic University, Hong Kong, PRC
[2] Centre for Innovation Programmes for Adolescents and Families,
The Hong Kong Polytechnic University, Hong Kong, PRC
[3]Kiang Wu Nursing College of Macau, Macau, PRC
[4]Department of Social Work, East China Normal University, Shanghai, PRC
[5]Division of Adolescent Medicine, Kentucky Children's Hospital,
University of Kentucky, Lexington, United States of America

ABSTRACT

Based on the responses of 275 Chinese adolescents experiencing economic disadvantage in Hong Kong, the relationships between family processes (including perceived parenting style, parental control, family functioning and parental sacrifice for children's education) and psychosocial competence were examined in this study. Results showed that parenting style, parental control, family functioning, and parental sacrifice for children's education were positively related to adolescent psychosocial competence. Regression analyses indicated that the family functioning, maternal control, and paternal sacrifice for children's education were significant predictors of psychosocial competence of

* Correspondence: Professor Daniel TL Shek, PhD, FHKPS, BBS, JP, Chair Professor of Applied Social Sciences, Faculty of Health and Social Sciences, Department of Applied Social Sciences, The Hong Kong Polytechnic University, Room HJ407, Core H, Hunghom, Hong Kong. E-mail: daniel.shek@polyu.edu.hk.

adolescents experiencing economic disadvantage. Theoretical and practical implications of the findings are discussed.

INTRODUCTION

There are theoretical and empirical concerns on the detrimental impacts of poverty on adolescent development. There is ample research on the impacts of poverty on adolescent psychological functioning (1-5). Theoretically, the "family stress model" of economic hardship has become the mainstream model for studying the impacts of poverty on adolescent development via family processes. The model addresses how parental distress and parenting behaviors mediate the effects of poverty on adolescent development (6,7).

Recently, researchers adopting the "family investment model" are concerned about how family resources and home environment affect child development in the context of poverty. Parents invest their time, energy, and money for their children's up-bringing. At the same time, children with more human capital would enhance their cognitive ability, academic achievement, and social-emotional well-being (7). However, for families in poverty, cognitive and psychological development of children is usually restricted with limited income available for investment.

With reference to the existing theories and research findings, one may have the following questions: while economically disadvantaged adolescents face debilitating psychological or behavioral problems, why do some adapt so well? Where does their driving force come from? This has been the concern of researchers and theorists in the field of resilience. Comparatively, little research was conducted on the processes that contribute to resilience and competence of adolescents experiencing poverty (8). McLoyd et al. (9) pointed out that there was "a dearth of research about contributors to positive adaptation in the context of socioeconomic disadvantage" (p. 446). Among the studies on resilience, Garmezy (10) suggested three categories of protective factors that moderated the influences of poverty: 1) personality/dispositional features, such as self-esteem, locus of control, self-efficacy, optimum; 2) affectional ties within the families, such as cohesion, warmth, shared values, consistency of rules, and support from adults; and 3) availability of external support systems such as schools, churches and caring agencies. Echoing these suggestions, other studies also indicated that familial qualities and processes are important in buffering the impacts of poverty for economically disadvantaged adolescents (11-13). In particular, the study of the relational world-view of Native Americans by Cross (14) gives insight on how family resilience is important in protecting family members from risks and vulnerabilities, as well as building up resilience of individuals in face of adversity. Cross (14) suggested that family resilience was enhanced through the process of parenting, as families passed on their beliefs, culture, values, and skills to their children. What the parents did to cope with the changes was simply "parent[ing] for resiliency" (14).

Several limitations were found in the studies concerning the relationships between family processes and adolescent psychosocial competence in economically disadvantaged families. First, it was found that a large majority of research employed the "deficiency" paradigm which focused on the detrimental impacts of poverty on internalizing and externalizing outcomes of economically disadvantaged adolescents (1-5). As such, studies employing "positive development" perspective on understanding the family strengths as well as adolescent competence lagged far behind. Criticizing "deficiency" models in research, Burton and Jarrett (15) suggested that youth are "erroneously assigned aberrant attributions when in fact their behaviors represent a cadre of actions that fit contextual demands" (p. 1118). In particular, research studying family characteristics and processes that build up adolescent resilience against adversity is lacking. Smith and Carlson (16) commented that "while there is ample research on the role of social support in mediating stress in adults, there is comparatively less research on social support for child and adolescent adjustment" (p. 239).

Second, many Chinese researches on family processes employed the conceptualization of Western theories. Shek (17) questioned the compatibility of Western theories and research findings when applied to Chinese people, especially Western family concepts and theories built on individualistic values that may be contradictory to the collectivistic ideology of Chinese families. Chao (18) also criticized Western descriptions of Chinese parenting for being "rather ethnocentric and misleading" (p. 1111). Yang (19) argued that unquestioning borrowing of Western concepts and tools results in inhibition of native values, views, and ways of thinking. There is an urgent need to develop indigenous Chinese conception of family processes and parenting. Chao and Tseng (20) identified three central themes for Asian parenting: centrality of the family and family interdependence, parental control and strictness, and fostering of educational achievement of children. Thus, the conceptions of family processes should be culturally specific and indigenously sensitive in non-western cultures.

The problems of conceptualization and indigenisation of psychosocial competence and family processes bring forth the problems of measurement tools. There was a severe lack of psychosocial assessment tools in the Chinese culture (21,22). Hence, indigenous measurement tools that accurately capture Chinese conceptions of psychosocial competence and family processes are indispensable.

Another limitation is that the impact of family processes on adolescent development is a complex process that may involve more than one pathway (23). Furthermore, it is unexplored which family process, if any, is comparatively more important for enhancing adolescent psychosocial competence than the others. To solve the problem, Shek (24) suggested that "different aspects of parenting can reveal the complex nature of the linkage between parenting and adolescent psychological well-being" (p. 273).

Last but not least, the differential roles of fathers and mothers in the adjustment of Chinese adolescents experiencing economic disadvantage remain to be clarified. While, there were inconsistent research findings on the differential roles of fathers and mothers in poor families (25), the research findings of differential roles of fathers and mothers in relation to the adjustment of Chinese adolescents were also found to be equivocal. The traditional view of "strict fathers, kind mothers" (26) in Chinese culture is challenged (27,28).

Based on the social capital theory of the family, Coleman (29,30) suggested that family influences on individual's behaviors have three distinct components – financial, human, and social capital. In the family system, financial capital represents the wealth or income of the families. Human capital is the potential parents provide for a cognitive environment of the children. Social capital is the set of resources that family members access through social ties which represent "the quantity and quality of networks that connect the children with resources of the parents" (31, p. 227).

In addition, Coleman (29) highlighted three essential forms of social capital: 1) obligations and expectations of family members, 2) information channels, and 3) norms and effective sanctions. In a family system, they represent parenting strategies, relational qualities among family members, communication patterns within the family, and family norms. Gofen (32) further elaborated the conceptualization of family capital as "the ensemble of means, strategies, and the resources embodied in the family's way of life that influences the future of their children" (32, p. 115).

There are different family processes that constitute social capital for adolescent development. Parenting style, the process of how the parents socialize their children, is considered as the fundamental one (33). There is empirical support on the relationships between parenting styles and adolescent psychosocial adjustment (8,16,34,35).

An affective and supportive family climate is essential for psychosocial development of the adolescents. Family functioning is an important family process that describes the quality of family life at the systemic level (36) and influences strongly adolescent psychological well-being (36-39). However, it should be noted that there are differences in the cultural norms for "healthy" family functioning between Western and Chinese societies. Based on a study to find out the attributes of happy families in Hong Kong, the results showed that Chinese parents and their children regarded the absence of conflict, interpersonal harmony, mutuality, connectedness, and positive parent-adolescent relationships as major attributes of happy family (40). Emotional expressiveness and communication are less likely to be regarded as attributes of a happy family, but they are important attributes in defining "healthy" family functioning in the Western societies (41-43).

It is noteworthy that parental control and parental sacrifice are distinctive features of Chinese parenting (20,44). While parental sacrifice involves parents' investment and involvement in children's education, parental control sets family standards and expectations for the children to follow. On the one hand, both parental control and parental sacrifice establish clear expectations and shared family standards which would help to build resilience and competence of adolescents. On the other hand, pressure, shame, and guilt would result if adolescents fail to reach the parents' standard and expectations. This would bring adverse effects on adolescents' emotional adjustment and self-development. Unfortunately, research on the relationships between parental control, parental sacrifice and psychosocial competence of Chinese adolescents experiencing economic disadvantage is scarce. Thus, it is interesting and illuminating to study the relationships of a diversified set of family processes of parenting style, parental control, parental sacrifice for children's education, and family functioning with adolescent psychosocial competence in Chinese economically disadvantaged families.

Two research questions were formulated in this study. The first question is: Are there any relationships between family processes and psychosocial competence of economically disadvantaged adolescents? Based on social capital theory of the family (29,30) and the family process models (34-36), seven hypotheses were formulated in this study. It was hypothesized that: a) more positive paternal and maternal parenting styles would be related to higher psychosocial competence of adolescents (Hypothesis 1a and 1b); b) higher levels of paternal and maternal control would be associated with higher psychosocial competence of adolescents (Hypothesis 1c and 1d); c) higher levels of paternal and maternal sacrifice for children's education would be associated with higher adolescent psychosocial competence (Hypothesis 1e and 1f); and d) a higher level of family functioning would be associated with higher psychosocial competence of adolescents (Hypothesis 1g).

The second research question is: What is the relative contribution of family processes to psychosocial competence of Chinese adolescents experiencing economic disadvantage? As research on this area is virtually non-existent, it is theoretically and practically important to explore the relative importance of dyadic family processes and systemic family functioning in predicting adolescent psychosocial competence.

OUR STUDY

A cross-sectional quantitative study was designed and purposeful sampling was employed. Adolescents from intact families at ages of 11 to 16 experiencing economic disadvantage were invited to participate in the study. The concept of relative poverty was adopted in the study, with 50% of monthly median domestic household income according to the Hong Kong Population By-census 2006 selected as the poverty threshold. The economically disadvantaged families were identified and recruited by children and youth service centers, school social work services, and community centers across Hong Kong wide. Finally, there were 276 families participating in the study. There was one adolescent questionnaire that was found to be invalid; thus 275 adolescent questionnaires were analyzed.

Either the first author or trained social workers conducted the data collection. Adolescents were given explanations about the purpose of the research, the procedure of data collection, the rights of respondents to voluntarily participate and withdraw from the study, as well as the use of the data in the study. Consent forms were given to adolescents and their parents. Signed informed consent from both parents and adolescents was sought. Adolescents were requested to complete the Adolescent Questionnaire which contained several scales, including Paternal Parenting Style Scale (APPS), Maternal Parenting Style Scale (AMPS), Chinese Paternal Control Scale (APCS), Chinese Maternal Control Scale (AMCS), Chinese Family Assessment Inventory (AFAI), Paternal Sacrifice for Children's Education Scale (APSA), Maternal Sacrifice for Children's Education Scale (AMSA), and the seven subscales of Chinese Positive Youth Development Scale (CPYDS). The questionnaire was administered in a self-administered format. Adolescents took around 35 minutes to complete the questionnaires.

There were 134 boys (48.7%) and 141 girls (51.3%) participating in the study. The ratio was close to that of the profile based on secondary schools (51.3: 48.7) in Hong Kong according to the 2006 Population By-census. The mean age of the adolescents was 13.56 (*SD* = 1.54), with the mean of boys and girls at 13.40 (*SD* = 1.60) and 13.71 (*SD* = 1.47) respectively. There were 18 adolescents (6.5%) studying in Primary Five or below (Grade 5 and below), 47 (17.1%) in Primary Six (Grade 6), 63 (22.9%) in Secondary One (Grade 7), 46 (16.7%) in Secondary Two (Grade 8), 42 (15.3%) in Secondary Three (Grade 9), 28 (10.2%) in Secondary Four (Grade 10), and 29 (10.5%) in Secondary Five and above (Grade 11 and above). Regarding duration of stay in Hong Kong, 144 adolescents (52.4%) were born in Hong Kong, and 74 (27.0%) had resided in Hong Kong for more than 7 years. But still, 24 (8.7%) adolescents had resided in Hong Kong for less than 3 years.

As for the family profile, the mean ages of the fathers and mothers were 49.94 (*SD* = 9.28) and 42.18 (*SD* = 4.97) respectively. Most fathers were born in Hong Kong (n = 98, 35.6%) or had resided in Hong Kong for more than 20 years (n = 115, 41.8%), whereas the highest percentage of mode of duration of stay of mothers in Hong Kong was between 6 and 10 years (n = 103, 37.5%). Regarding the educational standard of fathers and mothers, a majority were of low educational standard, with 205 fathers (74.5%) and 204 mothers

(74.2%) completing junior secondary level or lower. There were 211 (76.7%) fathers who had a job, 30 (10.9%) were unemployed, and 26 (9.5%) had retired. A high proportion of mothers were housewives (n = 199, 72.4%). The average number of children in the families was 2.34 (*SD* = .90). There were 96 families receiving Comprehensive Social Security Assistance from the Government, representing 34.8% of the sample.

Instruments

Paternal Parenting Style Scale (APPS) and Maternal Parenting Style Scale (AMPS). Based on the framework of Maccoby and Martin (45) and parenting assessment work of Lamborn et al. (34), Shek (46) developed a modified version of the Paternal/Maternal Parenting Style Scale (APPS/AMPS). There are two subscales: 1) Paternal/Maternal Demandingness Scale (PDEM/MDEM) assessing demandingness of the father and mother towards the child's behaviors; and 2) Paternal/Maternal Responsiveness Scale (PRES/MRES) assessing responsiveness of the father and mother to the child's behaviors. There are 7 items in the Demandingness Scale and 13 items in the Responsiveness Scale. The scales were found valid and reliable in the Chinese culture with internal consistency, test-retest reliability, and concurrent validity (46,47). Higher levels on the Paternal/Maternal Parenting Style Scale indicate more positive parental attributes. Reliability analyses showed that both APPS and AMPS had satisfactory reliability in this study (α =.856 and .834, respectively).

Chinese Paternal Control Scale (APCS) and Chinese Maternal Control Scale (AMCS). Based on a review of the literature, Shek (48,49) developed a twelve-item Chinese Paternal/Maternal Control Scale to assess control based on indigenous Chinese cultural beliefs. Adolescents were requested to rate the degree of agreement with each item on a 4-point scale ranging from "Strongly agree" to "Strongly disagree". Examples of the items are "My father expects me to be mature (*sheng xing*)"; "My father expects me to have good behavior so that I will not bring dishonor to the family (*you ru jia sheng*)". The APCS and AMCS showed internal consistency and divergent validity (49). The total score of the items in each scale is an indicator of the degree of parental control based on Chinese concepts, with a higher score indicating a higher level of Chinese parental control. Reliability analyses showed that both APCS and AMCS had satisfactory reliability in this study (α = .870 and .876, respectively).

Paternal/Maternal Sacrifice for Children's Education Scale (APSA/AMSA). Based on the literature on family investment (7), family capital (29,30), and parental involvement in children's education (41,50), as well as qualitative findings from focus groups of parents and adolescents respectively, an indigenous scale assessing parental sacrifice for children's education was developed (51). The scale was developed with 23 items measuring dimensions of sacrifice in terms of financial resources, time spent on children's education, reorganization of daily routine, sacrifice of lifestyle and aspiration, and shielding from worries. Participants were requested to rate the degree of agreement with each item on a 6-point Likert scale ranging from "Strongly agree" to "Strongly disagree". Examples of the items are "To fulfill my educational needs, my father eats and wears less"; "Even if/when my father is tired, he tries his best to understand my school life". Both APSA and AMSA showed internal consistency, divergent validity and factorial validity in validation study (52). Higher scores indicate greater parental sacrifice for children's education. Reliability analyses showed that both APSA and AMSA had high reliability in this study (α = .938 and .942, respectively).

The Chinese Family Assessment Instrument (AFAI). The AFAI is an indigenous 33-item self-report instrument to assess family functioning in Chinese populations. The AFAI has five subscales – mutuality, communication, conflict and harmony, parental concern, and parental control. Higher scores indicate higher level of family functioning. Shek and his colleagues (53,54) performed a series of validity studies that examined the factor structure, reliability, concurrent, and discriminant validity of AFAI and showed that that the scale was a valid and reliable measure of family functioning in the Chinese community. The scale was demonstrated to have excellent reliability in this study (α = .949).

Chinese Positive Youth Development Scale (CPYDS). Shek et al. (55) developed a 90-item Chinese Positive Youth Development Scale (CPYDS) that contains 15 aspects of positive youth development. Among the 15 aspects, 7 subscales measuring the psychosocial competence of adolescents were used in this study: 1) The resilience subscale (RE) is a six-item subscale that measures the capacity to adapt to changes and stressful events in healthy and adaptive ways. Some items were modelled after the items of the *Chinese Beliefs about Adversity Scale* (56). 2) The cognitive competence subscale (CC) is a six-item subscale that measures cognitive skills such as problem solving and goal setting, with some items modelled after the Chinese version of the *Social Problem-solving Inventory* (57). 3) The self-determination subscale (SD) is a 5-item subscale that measures the sense of autonomy, independent thinking and self-advocacy. 4) The self-efficacy subscale (SE) is a 2-item subscale that measures skills for coping and mastery. 5) The spirituality subscale (SP) is a 7-item subscale that measures sense of purpose and meaning in life, hope, and beliefs in a higher power. The items were modelled after the *Purpose in Life Questionnaire* (58). 6) The "beliefs in the future" subscale (BF) is a 3-item subscale that measures the ability to develop future goals and choices. 7) The "clear and positive identity" subscale (CPI) is a 7-item subscale that measures the development of healthy identity formation and achievement. The CPYDS showed acceptable internal consistency, criterion-related validity, construct validity and convergent validity with scores of Thriving Scale (TH), Life Satisfaction Scale (LIFE) and Perceived Academic Performance Scale (PAP) as well as discriminant validity with scores of Substance Abuse Scale (SA), Delinquency Scale (DE) and Behavioral Intention Scale (BI) (54). A Short-Form of CPYDS was developed with 3, 3, 3, 3, 3, 3 and 2 items for RE, CC, SD, SP, BF, CPI and SE respectively. The scale was demonstrated to have excellent reliability in this study (α = .941).

FINDINGS

To analyse the relationships between family processes and adolescent psychosocial competence, Pearson correlation analyses were performed. In order to decrease the chance of committing Type I error, a conservative alpha level based on Bonferroni correction (alpha = .05/7, i.e. .007) was adopted.

Before assessing the correlation between demographic variables and adolescent perception of family processes and psychosocial competence, it was found that perceived paternal parenting style (APPS) was significantly associated with age of adolescents (r = -

.275, $p < .001$) and educational level of adolescents ($r = -.224$, $p < .001$), suggesting that older, more educated adolescents had lower endorsement of perceived positive paternal parenting styles. The amount of overlap on the correlation of APPS on age and educational level of adolescents were 7.56%, and 5.02% of the variance. Thus, partial correlations of APPS scores by age of adolescents and educational levels of adolescents were carried out. Similarly, perceived maternal parenting style (AMPS) was significantly associated with age of adolescents ($r = -.303$, $p < .001$) and educational level of adolescents ($r = -.246$, $p < .001$), suggesting that older, more educated adolescents had less endorsement of positive maternal parenting style. The amount of overlap on the correlation of AMPS on age and educational level of adolescents were 9.18%, and 6.05% of the variance. Therefore, partial correlations of AMPS scores by age of adolescents and educational level of adolescents were recommended.

Moreover, adolescents' perception of family functioning (AFAI) was significantly related to their status of receiving CSSA ($r = -.216$, p < .001), suggesting that those families receiving CSSA would have relatively lower family functioning perceived by adolescents. Because the amount of overlap on the correlation of AFAI and status of CSSA recipient was 4.67% of the variance, partial correlation of AFAI scores by status of CSSA recipient would be performed.

Regarding Research Question 1, Hypotheses 1a and 1b were supported as perceived positive endorsement of paternal and maternal parenting styles were associated significantly with psychosocial competence of economically disadvantaged adolescents, with Pearson's *r* at .332 ($p < .001$) and .298 ($p < .001$) respectively. The effect size was medium. The relationships remained significant when age and educational level of adolescents were controlled. Besides, perceived paternal and maternal control was also correlated with psychosocial competence of adolescents, with Pearson's *r* at .327 ($p < .001$) and .345 ($p < .001$) respectively. The effect size was medium. Hypotheses 1c and 1d were thus supported. Furthermore, perceived paternal and maternal sacrifice for children's education were associated significantly with psychosocial competence of economically disadvantaged adolescents, with Pearson's r of .381 ($p < .001$) and .281 ($p < .001$) respectively. The effect sizes were between medium to large. Hypotheses 1e and 1f were supported.

Finally, it was found that family functioning was associated significantly with their psychosocial competence, with Pearson's r of .569 ($p < .001$). The effect size was large. With the control of status of CSSA recipients, the value of Pearson's *r* was reduced to .556 ($p < .001$), which still indicated significant correlation. Table 1 shows the correlations between the family processes and psychosocial competence of adolescents experiencing economic disadvantage.

Regarding the contribution of different family processes to psychosocial competence, hierarchical regression analyses were performed. Demographic variables (age and educational levels of adolescents, status of CSSA recipients) and family processes (paternal and maternal parenting styles, paternal and maternal control, paternal and maternal sacrifice for children's education, and family functioning) were entered into hierarchical blocks.

It was identified that perceived family functioning ($\beta = .499$, $p < .001$), maternal control ($\beta = .196$, $p < .01$), and paternal sacrifice for children's education ($\beta = .166$, $p < .05$) strongly predicted psychosocial competence of adolescents. The change of R^2 in Step 2 was .354, indicating that the overall family processes have substantial influences on enhancing psychosocial competence of adolescents experiencing economic disadvantage.

Table 2 shows the hierarchical regression analyses of adolescent psychosocial competence in economically disadvantaged families. Figure 1 shows the prediction of different family processes for psychosocial competence of adolescents.

Table 1. Correlations between relative family processes and psychosocial competence perceived by adolescents experiencing economic disadvantage

		Adolescents						
		Perceived parental parenting style		Perceived parental control		Perceived family functioning	Perceived parental sacrifice	
		APPS	AMPS	APCS	AMCS	AFAI	APSA	AMSA
Adolescents	PYD	.332*** (.315***)[a]	.298*** (.278***)[a]	.327***	.345***	.569*** (.556***)[b]	.381***	.281***

Note 1. *** $p < .001$.

Note 2. [a] The number in parentheses was the correlation coefficient calculated after age and educational level of adolescents were controlled. [b] The number in parentheses was the correlation coefficient calculated after status of CSSA recipients was controlled.

Note 3. APPS= Perceived Paternal Parenting Style Scale. AMPS= Perceived Maternal Parenting Style Scale. APCS= Perceived Paternal Control Scale. AMCS= Perceived Maternal Control Scale. APSA= Perceived Paternal Sacrifice for Children's Education Scale. AMSA= Perceived Maternal Sacrifice for Children's Education Scale. AFAI= Perceived Family Assessment Inventory. PYD= Chinese Positive Youth Development Scale (with 7 subscales selected).

Table 2. Hierarchical regression analyses of psychosocial competence of adolescents experiencing economic disadvantage

	Step 1 (β)	Step 2 (β)
Age of adolescents	-.097	-.079
Educational level of adolescents	-.011	.075
CSSA status	-.145*	-.029
Paternal parenting style		-.109
Maternal parenting style		-.018
Paternal control		.041
Maternal control		.196**
Paternal sacrifice for children's education		.166*
Maternal sacrifice for children's education		-.018
Family functioning		.499***
F	3.120	16.703
R^2	.033	.388
ΔR^2		.354

β = Standardized regression coefficient.

*$p < .05$, ** $p < .01$, *** $p < .001$.

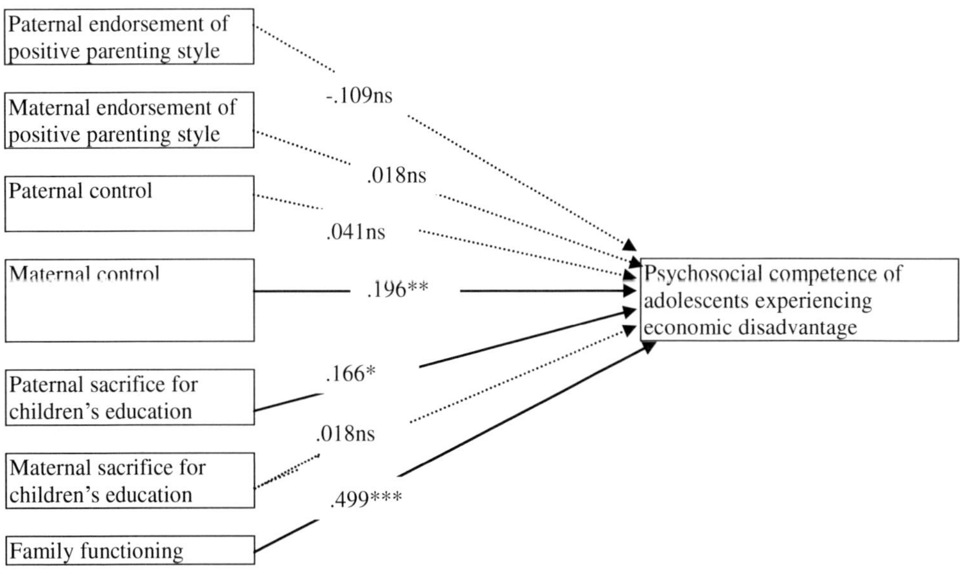

*p < .05, **p < .01, ***p <.001, ns=not significant.
Note. Solid line = significant relationship; Dotted line = non-significant relationship.

Figure 1. Predictions of different family processes on psychosocial competence of adolescents experiencing economic disadvantage.

Discussion

The present findings support the social capital theory of the family (29,30) as well as family process models that positive parental qualities such as positive parenting style, parental management and supervision, parental sacrifice and involvement, warm and stable family environment are associated with better psychological well-being of adolescents living in poverty (8,23,59). The findings also echoed the resilience literature that family processes serve as protective factors against the adverse effects of poverty (10-13,35). The present findings showed that all measured family processes (parenting style, parental control, family functioning, parental sacrifice) perceived by adolescents were significantly related to psychosocial competence of adolescents. Among the relationships of various family processes and adolescent psychosocial competence, it was found that the effect of family functioning was the greatest. The other family processes also had the strength of effect ranging from medium to high level. The present findings strongly suggest that parents do "make a difference" in building psychosocial competence and resilience of economically disadvantaged adolescents. Among the family processes, it was found that family functioning remarkably influenced adolescent psychosocial competence. Maternal control and paternal sacrifice for children's education also significantly predicted adolescent psychosocial competence.

The literature on resilience suggests that a warm and stable family environment with affectional familial relationships serves as an important familial buffer of poor adolescents facing adversity (10,16,35). From a family perspective, resilient poor families demonstrated high levels of warmth, affection, emotional support for one another and sustained family rules, routines and shared core values (60,61). There is also empirical support that positive family functioning was related to better adolescent adjustment in low socio-economic context (37-39). Thus, it is unquestionable that family functioning is an important predictor of enhanced adolescent psychosocial competence. However, we should bear in mind that the relationships between family functioning and adolescent psychological well-being were found to be bi-directional in nature in longitudinal studies (62). As this research is cross-sectional in research design, this is a limitation to be addressed in future studies.

Maternal control was another significant predictor of adolescent psychosocial competence. There is a concern that since shame strategy has been an indigenous Chinese socialization practice (63,64), guilt and shame would arise if adolescents could not meet mothers' expectations and standards. The stresses and emotional disturbance may result in poor psychosocial competence of adolescents. However, the findings showed that maternal control predicted adolescent psychosocial competence, a finding which suggests that clear expectations from and shared similar standards with their mothers help adolescents to develop clear and positive identity, self-efficacy, and resilience, rather than causing stresses, shame and guilt that may disrupt adolescent psychosocial competence. Moreover, clear family expectations and standards would help family members to cultivate a sense of coherence that crisis could be manageable and meaningful (43), which are essential for economically disadvantaged adolescents to develop resilience in facing adversity. As mothers spent more time in monitoring their children and were more involved in the parenting roles, maternal control was found to be more salient in influencing the psychosocial competence of adolescents. In addition, it was found that the emphasis of interdependence in the Chinese family system was more salient in mother-child relationships, as Chinese mothers emphasized the relational goals of fostering enduring mother-child relationships and sharing of love and affection (20). Thus, adolescents were more sensitive and responsive to mother-child relationships.

Last but not least, paternal sacrifice for children's education influenced psychosocial competence of adolescents. Paternal sacrifice for children's education implies the love, expectation and support of the fathers for the adolescents, which is important for enhancing adolescent psychosocial competence, and essentially helps adolescents develop clear future orientation and positive self-identity.

It is interesting to identify different roles of fathers and mothers in enhancing the psychosocial competence of economically disadvantaged adolescents. Fathers, as breadwinners, are responsible for protecting family members and striving for family resources for maintenance of family daily necessities and adolescent development. This is particularly important for poor families, as fathers put extraordinary effort into striving for financial resources and make more sacrifice for their children's development with these scarce resources. Thus, adolescents perceived paternal sacrifice for children's education as an expression of fathers' love, support and contribution to the families that enhanced psychosocial competence of adolescents. Mothers, on the other hand, are mainly responsible for child-rearing roles such as caring, nurturing and monitoring children's behaviors in the families. As the child-rearing role is central to mothers' responsibilities, maternal control was considered a significant predictor of psychosocial competence of adolescents. The findings echo with the cultural inclination of "*Nan zhu wai, nu zhu nei*" (men manage things outside the family, whereas women manage things inside the family) in Chinese community.

However, the strong traditional discourse of "strict fathers, kind mothers" (26) in Chinese culture that fathers are regarded as "harsh disciplinarians" and mothers are kind and affectionate (65) is challenged. The differential roles of fathers and mothers point to a "strict mother, kind father" thesis (27,28) with mothers' contribution to adolescent psychosocial competence focusing on control and monitoring, whereas fathers' contribution focuses on sacrifice and support to the families. Nevertheless, the differential contributions of fathers and mothers to building adolescents' psychosocial competence are illuminating for us to understand the complex family processes of poor families.

There are theoretical and practical implications of the study. First, the present study employed the "positive youth development" paradigm on studying the family processes that enhanced psychosocial competence of economic disadvantaged adolescents, which sheds new light on helping the adolescents to beat the odds of poverty, and resolving the problems of intergenerational poverty. Contrary to the mainstream "deficiency" paradigm that focused on the detrimental effects of poverty on the families and adolescents (1-5), the findings bring important additions to the literature. Second, the study underscores the importance of indigenous conceptualization of theoretical models that fit the unique Chinese context. The concepts of parental control, family functioning and parental sacrifice for children's education were indigenously developed in the Chinese context where collectivistic orientation and Confucian thought were stressed. The findings suggest that maternal control and parental sacrifice for children's education, which are the distinctive features of Chinese parenting practices (20,43), are influential family processes that enhance psychosocial competence of adolescents experiencing economic disadvantage. The study demonstrates the importance of employment of indigenous Chinese concepts in the theorisation and development of Chinese family models.

Third, different family processes were studied in their relationships with adolescent psychosocial competence in the context of poverty. To conceptualize the complexity of family processes and family relationships, dyadic (father-adolescent, mother-adolescent) family processes including parenting style, parental control, parental sacrifice for children's education, as well as systemic family processes of family functioning were explored. The family processes provide us important information on the different roles and contributions of fathers and mothers in parenting their children, and the family relationsips address the interdependence among family relationships. In view of paucity of studies that examine both dyadic and systemic family processes in association with adolescent psychosocial competence, the present study was considered pioneering in the Chinese community.

Fourth, the findings suggest that family processes, family functioning in particular, are essential predictors for enhancing psychosocial competence of adolescents. These provide important cues on family intervention in helping economically disadvantaged families. Instead of taking a residual model approach on providing tangible support for the families, or putting emphasis solely on the adolescents in overcoming the odds of poverty, a family-based intervention approach to help the economically disadvantaged families is urged. Family-life education, emotional support for parents, parenting enhancement programs, etc., would be necessary for parents to cultivate the psychosocial competence of adolescents.

Fifth, the present findings clearly show that besides positive youth development programs which attempt to promote psychosocial competencies in young people, family is another important level for intervention. In the specific context of Hong Kong, there are researches showing that positive youth development programs such as the Project P.A.T.H.S. are beneficial to the holistic development of adolescent (66-72). While such findings are important as far as school-based programs are concerned, the present study suggests that family-based programs are also important.

Last but not least, the different roles of fathers and mothers in enhancing adolescent psychosocial competence imply a call for gender-sensitive practice in family intervention of economically disadvantaged families. The different roles of fathers and mothers entail different needs of fathers and mothers. Fathers, responsible for mobilizing family resources for the families, may experience great pressure when their wages are minimal and fluctuating. This may weaken their perceived contributions to the family and thus induce psychological stresses. On the other hand, mothers take up more parental roles in monitoring and control, apart from the conventional expectations of caring and nurturing. As "higher behavioral control would be physically and psychologically taxing for mothers" (27, p. 679), mothers would shoulder most burden in taking up dual roles of monitoring and nurturing their children. The strains and stresses of performing family roles may affect the psychological well-being of fathers and mothers, and may cause marital conflict. Social workers and clinical practitioners should be sensitive to the different roles of fathers and mothers and address their psychological and parenting needs.

There are several limitations of the present study. First, the limitation of purposeful sampling should be recognized. As adolescents recruited were not randomly sampled, generalizability of the findings may be limited. Second, the cross-sectional design in this study has the inherent problem in inferring cause-and-effect relationships. For instance, it was found that the relationships between family functioning and adolescent psychological well-being were bi-directional in nature in longitudinal studies (61). Because the present study was cross-sectional in nature, the causal relationships between family functioning and adolescent psychological well-being could not be adequately assessed. Hence, a longitudinal research design is recommended in future studies. Third, as the assessment of family processes was based on the self-reported questionnaires, the findings may only represent the perceptions of the "insiders". Wampler and Halverson (73) pointed out that quantitative measurement is weakest in "capturing the complexity of family life" (p. 189). It would be more illuminating to include the observation data in real-life settings from the "outsiders" view so that a more comprehensive picture of family processes can be obtained.

Fourth, the information collected was based on the adolescents only. Day et al. (74) argued that considering response from just one person in family research provides "a very limited basis for extrapolating a sequence of events that may lead to a certain decision or interactional style" (p. 110). Information from multiple informants such as parents would be desirable. Last but not least, as the findings presented in the study were based on economically disadvantaged adolescents in Hong Kong, there is a need to assess the generalizability of the findings in different Chinese communities (e.g. mainland China) and Chinese people living in non-Chinese contexts (e.g. Chinese-Americans).

Despite these limitations, the present findings can be regarded as pioneering and stimulating in view of the paucity of research in studying the relationships between different family processes and psychosocial competence of Chinese adolescents experiencing economic disadvantage. Essentially, the study is an active and constructive response to McLoyd et al.'s (9) comment that there is "a dearth of research about contributors to positive adaptation [of adolescents] in the context of socioeconomic disadvantage" (p. 446). Similarly, as there are very few studies examining quality of life in Chinese adolescents experiencing economic disadvantage (21), the present findings are an important addition to the literature.

REFERENCES

[1] Bolger KE, Patterson CJ, Thompson WW, Kupersmidt JB. Psychosocial adjustment among children experiencing persistent and intermittent family economic hardship. Child Dev 1995;66(4):1107-29.
[2] Conger RD, Conger KJ, Elder GH Jr., Lorenz FO, Simons RL, Whitbeck LB. A family process model of economic hardship and adjustment of early adolescent boys. Child Dev 1992;63(3):526-41.
[3] Conger RD, Conger KJ, Elder GH Jr., Lorenz FO, Simons RL, Whitbeck LB. Family economic stress and adjustment of early adolescent girls. Dev Psychol 1993;29(2):206-19.
[4] Shek DTL. Family life quality and emotional quality of life in Chinese adolescents with and without economic disadvantage. Soc Indic Res 2007;80(2):393-410.
[5] Shek DTL. Economic disadvantage, perceived family life quality and emotional well-being in Chinese adolescents: A longitudinal studies. Soc Indic Res 2008;85(2):169-89.
[6] Conger RD, Conger KJ. Understanding the processes through which economic hardship influences families and children. In: Crane DR, Heaton TB, eds. Handbook of families and poverty. Thousand Oaks, LA: Sage, 2008:64-81.
[7] Conger RD, Donnellan MB. An interactionist perspective on the socioeconomic context of human development. Annu Rev Psychol 2007;58:175-99.
[8] Shek DTL. The relation of parental qualities to psychological well-being, school adjustment and problem behavior in Chinese adolescents with economic disadvantage. Am J Fam Ther 2002;30: 215-30.
[9] McLoyd VC, Kaplan R, Purtell KM, Bagley E, Hardaway CR, Smalls C. Poverty and socioeconomic disadvantage in adolescence. In Lerner RM, Steingberg L, eds. Handbook of adolescent psychology, Vol. 2: Contextual influences on adolescent development. Hoboken, NJ: John Wiley, 2009:444-91.
[10] Garmezy N. Children in poverty: Resilience despite risk. Psychiatry 1993;56(1):127-36.
[11] Masten AS, Best KM, Garmezy N. Resilience and development: Contributions from the study of children who overcome adversity. Dev Psychopathol 1990;2:425-44.
[12] Rutter M. Psychosocial resilience and protective mechanisms. In: Rolf J, Masten AS, Cicchetti D, Nüchterlein KH, Weintraub S, eds. Risk and protective factors in the development of psychopathology. UK: Cambridge Univ Press, 1990:181-214.
[13] Werner EE, Smith RS. Overcoming the odds: High risk children from birth to adulthood. Ithaca, NY: Cornell Univ Press, 1992.
[14] Cross TL. Understanding family resiliency from a relational world-view. In: McCubbin HI, Thompson EA, Thompson AI, Fromer JE, eds. Resiliency in ethnic minority families: Native and immigrant American families: Vol 1. Madison, WI: Univ Wisconsin System,1995:143-57.
[15] Burton L, Jarrett RL. In the mix, yet on the margins: The place of families in urban neighborhood and child development research. J Marriage Fam 2000;62(4):1114-35.
[16] Smith C, Carlson BE. Stress, coping, and resilience in children and youth. Soc Serv Rev 1997;71(2):231-56.
[17] Shek DTL. Chinese family research: Puzzles, progress, paradigms, and policy implications. J Fam Issues 2006;27(3):275-84.
[18] Chao RK. Beyond parental control and authoritarian parenting style: Understanding Chinese parenting through the cultural notion of training. Child Dev 1994;65(4):1111-9.
[19] Yang KS. Towards an indigenous Chinese psychology: A selective review of methodological, theoretical, and empirical accomplishments. Chinese J Psychol 1999;41(2):181-211.
[20] Chao RK, Tseng V. Parenting in Asians. In: Bornstein MH, ed. Handbook of parenting. Vol. 4: Social conditions and applied parenting. Mahwah, NJ: Lawrence Erlbaum, 2002:59-93.
[21] Shek DTL. Quality of life of Chinese people in a changing world. Soc Indic Res, 2010;95(3):357-61.

[22] Shek DTL, Lam MC, Tsoi KW. Evidence-based practice in Hong Kong. In: Thyer B, Kazi MAF, eds. International perspectives on evidence-based practice in social work. London: Venture Press, 2004:167-81.
[23] Bradley RH, Corwyn RF. Socioeconomic status and child development. Annu Rev Psychol 2002; 53:371-99.
[24] Shek DTL. Paternal and maternal influences on the psychological well-being of Chinese adolescents. Genet Soc Gen Psychol Monogr 1999;125(3):269-96.
[25] Harris KM, Marmer JK. Poverty, paternal involvement, and adolescent well-being. J Fam Issues 1996;17(5):614-40.
[26] Wilson RW. The moral state: A study of the political socialization of Chinese and American children. New York: Free Press, 1974.
[27] Shek DTL. A longitudinal study of perceived differences in parental control and parent-child relational qualities in Chinese adolescents in Hong Kong. J Adolesc Res 2007;22(2):156-88.
[28] Shek DTL. Perceived parental control and parent-child relational qualities in early adolescents in Hong Kong: Parent gender, child gender and grade differences. Sex Roles 2008;58:666-81.
[29] Coleman JS. Social capital in the creation of human capital. Am J Sociol 1988;94(Suppl 95):S95-S120.
[30] Coleman JS. Foundations of social theory. Cambridge, MA: Harvard Univ Press, 1990.
[31] Schlee BM, Mullis AK, Shriner M. Parents social and resource capital: Predictors of academic achievement during early childhood. Child Youth Serv Rev 2009;31(2):227-34.
[32] Gofen A. Family capital: How first-generation higher education students break the intergenerational cycle. Fam Relat 2009;58:104-20.
[33] Darling N, Steinberg L. Parenting style as context: An integrative model. Psychol Bull 1993;113(3):487-96.
[34] Lamborn SD, Mounts NS, Steinberg L, Dornbusch SM. Patterns of competence and adjustment among adolescents from authoritative, authoritarian, indulgent, and neglectful families. Child Dev 1991;62(5):1049-65.
[35] Wyman PA, Cowen EL, Work WC, Raoof A, Gribble PA, Parker GR, Wannon M. Interviews with children who experienced major life stress: Family and child attributes that predict resilient outcomes. J Am Acad Child Adolesc Psychiatry 1992;31(5):904-10.
[36] Shek DTL. A longitudinal study of perceived family functioning and adolescent adjustment in Chinese adolescents with economic disadvantage. J Fam Issues 2005;26(4):518-43.
[37] Bosma HA, Gerrits RS. Family functioning and identity status in adolescence. J Early Adolesc 1985;5(1):69-80.
[38] Shek DTL. Family functioning and psychological well-being, school adjustment, and problem behavior in Chinese adolescents with and without economic disadvantage. J Genet Psychol 2002;163(4):497-502.
[39] Street J, Harris-Britt A, Walker-Barnes C. Examining relationships between ethnic identity, family environment, and psychological outcomes for African American adolescents. J Child Fam Stud 2009;18(4):412-20.
[40] Shek DTL, Chan LK. Perceptions of the happy family in a Chinese context. J Youth Stud 1998;1:178-89.
[41] Epstein NB, Ryan CE, Bishop DS, Miller IW, Keitner GI. The McMaster Model: A view of healthy family functioning. In: Walsh F, ed. Normal family processes: Growing diversity and complexity. New York: Guilford, 2003:581-607.
[42] Quatman T. High functioning families: Developing a prototype. Fam Ther 1997;24(3):143-65.
[43] Walsh F, ed. Normal family processes: Growing diversity and complexity. New York: Guilford, 2003.
[44] Chao RK, Kaeochinda KF. Parental sacrifice and acceptance as distinct dimensions of parental support among Chinese and Filipino American adolescents. In: Russell ST, Crockett LJ, Chao RK, eds. Asian American parenting and parent–adolescent relationships, New York: Springer Sci Business Media, 2010:61-77.

[45] Maccoby EE, Martin JA. Socialization in the context of the family: Parent-child interaction. In: Mussen PH, series ed., Hetherington EM, vol. ed. Handbook of child psychology, Vol. 4: Socialization, personality, and social development. New York: Wiley, 1983:1-100.
[46] Shek DTL. Parenting characteristics and adolescent psychological well-being: A longitudinal study in a Chinese context. Genet Soc Gen Psychol Monogr 1999;125(1):27-44.
[47] Shek DTL. A longitudinal study of parenting and psychosocial adjustment among Chinese adolescents experiencing economic disadvantage. Int J Adolesc Med Health 2003;15(1):39-49.
[48] Shek DTL. Perceived parental control processes, parent-child relational qualities, and psychological well-being in Chinese adolescents with and without economic disadvantages. J Genet Psychol 2005;166(2):171-88.
[49] Shek DTL. Perceived parental control based on indigenous Chinese parental concepts in adolescents in Hong Kong. Am J Fam Ther 2007;35:123-37.
[50] Grolnick W, Benjet C, Kurowski C, Apostoleris N. Predictors of parent involvement in children's schooling. J Educ Psychol 1997;89(3):538-48.
[51] Leung, JTY, Shek DTL. "All I can do for my child" --- Development of the Chinese Parental Sacrifice for Child's Education Scale. Int J Disabil Hum Dev 2011;10(3):201-8.
[52] Leung, JTY, Shek DTL. Validation of the Chinese Parental Sacrifice for Child's Education Scale. Int J Disabil Hum Dev 2011;10(3):209-15.
[53] Shek DTL. Assessment of family functioning Chinese adolescents: The Chinese Family Assessment Instrument. In: Singh NN, Ollen-dick T, Singh AN, eds. International perspectives on child and adolescent mental health. Amsterdam, Netherlands: Elsevier, 2002:297-316.
[54] Siu AMH, Shek DTL. Psychometric properties of the Chinese Family Assessment Instrument in Chinese adolescents in Hong Kong. Adolescence 2005;40(160):817-30.
[55] Shek DTL, Siu AMH, Lee TY. The Chinese Positive Youth Development Scale: A validation study. Res Soc Work Pract 2007;17(3):380-91.
[56] Shek DTL. Beliefs about the causes of poverty in parents and adolescents experiencing economic disadvantage in Hong Kong. J Genet Psychol 2004;165(3):272-91.
[57] Siu AMH, Shek DTL. The Chinese version of the Social Problem-solving Inventory: Some initial results on reliability and validity. J Clin Psychol 2005;61(3):347-60.
[58] Shek DTL. Meaning in life and psychological well-being: An empirical study using the Chinese version of the Purpose in Life Questionnaire. J Genet Psychol 1992;153(2):185-200.
[59] Conger RD, Conger KJ. Resilience in Midwestern families: selected findings from the first decade of a prospective, longitudinal study. J Marriage Fam 2002;64(2):361-73.
[60] McCubbin HI, Thompson AI, McCubbin MA. Family assessment: Resiliency, coping and adaptation, Inventories for research and practice. Madison, WI: Univ Wisconsin Publishers, 1996.
[61] Seccombe K. 'Beating the odds' versus 'changing the odds': Poverty, resilience, and family policy. J Marriage Fam 2002;64(2):384-95.
[62] Shek DTL. A longitudinal study of the relationship between family functioning and adolescent psychological well-being. J Youth Stud 1998;1(2):195-209.
[63] Yang KS. The formation and change of Chinese personality: A cultural-ecological perspective. Acta Psychologica Taiwanica 1981; 23(1):39-55. [Chinese]
[64] Yang KS. Chinese personality and its change. In: Bond MH, ed. The psychology of Chinese people. Hong Kong: Oxford Univ Press, 1986:106-70.
[65] Shek DTL. Parenting characteristics and parent-adolescent conflict: A longitudinal study in the Chinese culture. J Fam Issues 2002;23(2):189-208.
[66] Shek DTL. Subjective outcome and objective outcome evaluation findings: Insights from a Chinese context. Res Soc Work Pract 2010;20(3):293-301.
[67] Shek DTL. Using students' weekly diaries to evaluate positive youth development programs: Are findings based on multiple studies consistent? Soc Indic Res 2010;95(3):475-87.
[68] Shek DTL, Ma CMS. Impact of the Project P.A.T.H.S. in the junior secondary school years: individual growth curve analyses. Sci World J 2011;10:253-66.
[69] Shek DTL, Merrick J, eds. Special issue: Positive youth development and training. Int J Adolesc Med Health 2010;22(3):341-447.

[70] Shek DTL, Ng CSM. Early identification of adolescents with greater psychosocial needs: an evaluation of the Project P.A.T.H.S. in Hong Kong. Int J Disabil Hum Dev 2010;9(4):291-9.

[71] Shek DTL, Yu L. Prevention of adolescent problem behavior: Longitudinal impact of the Project P.A.T.H.S. in Hong Kong. Sci World J 2011;11:546-67.

[72] Sun RCF, Shek DTL. Life satisfaction, positive youth development, and problem behaviour among Chinese adolescents in Hong Kong. Social Indic Res 2010;95(3):455-74.

[73] Wampler KS, Halverson CF Jr. Quantitative measurement in family research. In: Boss PG, Doherty WJ, LaRossa R, Schumm WR, Steinmetz SK, eds. Sourcebook of family theories and methods: A contextual approach. New York: Plenum Press, 1993:181-94.

[74] Day RD, Gavazzi S, Acock A. Compelling family processes. In: Thornton A. ed. The well-being of children and families – research and data needs. Ann Arbor, MI: Univ Michigan, 2001:103-26.

In: Chinese Adolescent Development ISBN: 978-1-62618-622-4
Editors: Daniel TL Shek, Rachel CF Sun, Joav Merrick © 2013 Nova Science Publishers, Inc.

Chapter 3

PARENTAL BELIEFS AND PARENTING CHARACTERISTICS OF CHINESE PARENTS EXPERIENCING ECONOMIC DISADVANTAGE IN HONG KONG

Janet TY Leung[1] and Daniel TL Shek[1,2,3,4,5]

[1]Department of Applied Social Sciences,
The Hong Kong Polytechnic University, Hong Kong, PRC
[2]Centre for Innovative Programmes for Adolescents and Families,
The Hong Kong Polytechnic University, Hong Kong, PRC
[3]Kiang Wu Nursing College of Macau, Macau, PRC
[4]Department of Social Work, East China Normal University,
Shanghai, PRC
[5]Division of Adolescent Medicine, Department of Pediatrics,
Kentucky Children's Hospital, University of Kentucky College of Medicine,
Lexington, Kentucky, US

ABSTRACT

Based on the responses of 550 Chinese parents experiencing economic disadvantage in Hong Kong, the relationships between parental beliefs (including Chinese cultural beliefs about adversity, attribution of children's success and failure to effort, and expectations of children's future) and parenting characteristics (indexed by parenting styles and parental control) were examined in this study. It was found that more positive parental child-specific beliefs, particularly parental expectations on children's future were associated with more positive parenting styles and stronger parental control in both fathers' and mothers' samples. Theoretical and practical implications of the findings are discussed.

INTRODUCTION

According to the ecological-cultural perspective, parenting practices are manifestations of parental belief systems (1). The cultural meanings embedded in a particular culture shape the parental beliefs systems and parenting goals, which in turn influence the parental roles and parenting practices (2). Thus, parental beliefs are important constructs that infuse and guide parents' actions. Beliefs enable individuals to cope with everyday challenges, generate parental behaviors in response to parenting demands, and serve as means to preserve parents' self-esteem, by setting standards for assessing and complying the parental roles and responsibilities (3).

Unfortunately, research on parental beliefs of poor families is minimal. Using the search terms of "poverty/economic disadvantage" and "parental belief", an advanced search of the PsycINFO in November 2011 for the period 1980-2011 showed that there were only 50 publications. Amongst these publications, there were only four pieces of work pertinent to the Chinese community. Similarly, computer search using search terms of "poverty/economic disadvantage" and "parental belief" of Social Work Abstracts in November 2011 for the period 1980-2011 showed that there was only one publication. The minimal research on parental beliefs of poor families may be due to the difficulties on theorization and conceptualization of belief systems, cultural-specificity of belief systems, and the lack of tools for measuring parental beliefs (4). As commented by Sigel and McGillicuddy-De Lisi (5), "a clear conception of beliefs [for parents] and theoretical explanations of how and why beliefs are effective are lacking" and that literature on beliefs "is superficial, poorly defined, and while often in face validity, it is sorely lacking in providing information about construct and content validity" (p. 497).

Apart from the severe lack of research on parental beliefs, there are other limitations pertinent to the research on understanding the relationships between parental beliefs and parenting characteristics in the context of poverty. First, there are problems on the conceptualization of parental beliefs. McGillicuddy-De Lisi and Sigel (3) highlighted four perspectives in the conceptualization of parental beliefs. They are attribution approaches, information-processing models, constructivist perspectives and transactional perspectives. It was found that the conceptions are not isomorphic with each other (3). However, there is very rare research examining different conceptions of parental beliefs in the beliefs system.

Second, according to the ecological perspective, culture has critical influence in laying down the ideological values, norms, and institutional patterns that make up the 'blueprints' for the ecology of human development (6). It affects the socialization process, parenting strategies and social adaptation. This is of critical importance in the Chinese context as the Chinese has her unique culture developed for over five thousand years under the influence of Confucianism, Taoism and Buddhism. Unfortunately, the cultural component of parental beliefs is often ignored. Leung (7) commented that "a dearth of theorizing and data on the beliefs systems of Chinese" (p. 262).

Similarly, many Chinese researches employed Western concepts of parenting characteristics in their studies, thus ignoring the cultural specificity in conceptualization of parenting. Shek (8) queried about the compatibility of Western theories and research findings when applied to Chinese people because Western family concepts and theories built on individualistic values may not be compatible with the collectivistic ideology of Chinese families. Chao (9) also criticized Western descriptions of Chinese parenting for being "rather ethnocentric and misleading" (p. 1111). Burton and Jerrett (10) further commented on the "lack of attention given to cultural and contextual perspectives of family processes" (p. 1128). Hence, there is an urgent need to develop indigenous Chinese conception of family processes and parenting.

Another limitation was that the relationships between parental beliefs and parenting characteristics were seldom explored. Miller (11) criticized that "the link between [parental] beliefs and [parenting] behaviors remains the most often discussed and least often studied topic in the parental beliefs literature" (p. 282). However, as mentioned before, parental beliefs may influence parenting strategies and parents' self-appraisal in fulfilling their parental roles, which in turn affect the cognitive, social and psychological development of children. The concern is more crucial for poor families as parental beliefs also affect the family's conceptualization of adversity and their coping mechanisms in the face of stress (12). The severe lack of research hinders theoretical model building in this area.

Methodologically speaking, the problem of conceptualization of parental beliefs and parenting characteristics brings forth the problems of measurement tools. As some researchers indicated, there was a severe lack of psychosocial assessment tools in the Chinese culture (13,14). In addition, indigenous measurement tools that accurately capture Chinese conceptions of parental beliefs and parenting characteristics are also rare in the literature.

Difficulties in capturing the complexity of parenting characteristics also constitute to a limitation of the related research. Conceptually, global parenting style and specific parenting practices are essential elements in constituting the central features of parenting (15). Shek (16) suggested that we should examine different aspects of parenting because they "can reveal the complex nature of the linkage between parenting and adolescent psychological well-being" (p. 273). As such, two separate measures of parenting should be used.

The final limitation of the related research is that there were few studies that captured the perspectives of both fathers and mothers. In many existing studies examining parenting characteristics, the role of primary caregivers, mostly the mothers, was the main focus (2,17-19) with the fathers usually not covered. The paucity of research on paternal roles in adolescent development may be due to difficulties in engaging fathers in research, as well as the public perception that fathers as "bread-winners" of the family were seldom involved in parenting their children. The negligence of fathers' roles is even more salient in poverty research. The physically demanding jobs as well as long and non-standard working hours usually create additional hurdles for economically disadvantaged fathers to be involved in research.

Among the very limited literature on parental beliefs in the context of poverty, two dimensions of parental beliefs, beliefs about adversity, and child-specific beliefs, are worth noting. Cultural beliefs contribute to the belief systems of parents about adversity by influencing how adversity is defined and conceptualized, as well as by shaping coping resources and behaviors (20). According to the resiliency model of family adjustment and adaptation, cultural beliefs have fundamental impacts that determine how the families give meaning to stressful life events and family struggles, as well as shape the family's responses and strategies (12). Parents with strong beliefs to overcome adversity tend to act positively in the face of difficulties and challenges, which in turn influences their children's development.

In Chinese communities, Lee (21) suggested that traditional beliefs help those in lower social-economic strata cope with stress from economic striving. However, he gave this a negative connotation that people use mythical explanations and manipulations of life's vicissitudes to cope with stress (21, p. 203). The mechanisms of how this explanation and manipulation buffers poor families' stress remained unexplored.

Recently, effort has been made in the conceptualization of Chinese cultural beliefs about adversity and exploration of relationships between endorsement of positive Chinese beliefs about adversity and psychological development of adolescents (20,22,23). Shek (22) classified Chinese cultural beliefs about adversity into two categories. The first category was positive beliefs about adversity which are cultural beliefs that emphasize the positive value of adversity and people's capacity to overcome it. These cultural beliefs are shaped by the Confucian emphasis on people's inner strengths and virtues, such as perseverance and tolerance. The second category of beliefs were negative beliefs about adversity are cultural beliefs that suggest impossibility and people's incapability to change adverse situations, as adversity may be due to fate or superstition. Some of these beliefs are also influenced by Buddhist and Taoist thoughts (22). However, relationships of Chinese cultural beliefs about adversity and family processes in poor families were unexplored.

Regarding child-specific parental beliefs, Eccles et al. (24) identified six child-specific parental beliefs that may influence parenting strategies which in turn affect children's motivation: 1) causal attributions for children's performance; 2) perceptions of the difficulty of a specific task; 3) expectations for their children's success, and confidence in their children's abilities; 4) beliefs about the value of the specific task; 5) differential achievement standards of fulfilling the task; and 6) beliefs about the external barriers to success (24, pp. 1058-1059).

Among these, parental expectation is one of the most significant factors predicting children's cognitive and psychological competence via parenting practices (25). A study of single-parent African American families found that mothers' developmental goals for children, indexed by being respectful, being well-educated, getting along with others and being well-behaved, influenced the academic and psychosocial competence of children through competence-promoting parenting practices (26).

Another parental child-specific belief that influences the development and achievement of their children is causal attributions for children's success and failure. Causal attributions directly impact parent's affective responses, parenting practices and involvement in children's activities, which in turn influences child and adolescent development (27-29). A study of 473 parents with children studying in sixth grade in public elementary schools showed that parental attribution of success to children's effort was positively related to the child's actual school achievement, through parental involvement in facilitating children's interests (28). On the contrary, parents who attributed success or failure to external characteristics (such as luck) might correlate with children's underachievement (29).

In the Chinese culture, effort in education is emphasized, as reflected by the sayings "*qin you gong, xi wu yi*" (reward lies ahead of diligence but nothing is gained by indolence), "*qin neng bu zhou*" (diligence is a means by which one makes up for one's dullness). Thus, according to Chinese cultural beliefs, effort is important in parental attribution of children's success and failure.

Regarding parenting characteristics, parenting style was regarded as the "fundamental" one (30). Parenting style is defined as "a constellation of attitudes toward the child that are communicated to the child and that, taken together, create an emotional climate in which the parents' behaviors are expressed. These behaviors include both the specific, goal-directed behaviors through which the parents perform their parental duties (to be referred as parenting practices) and non-goal-directed parental behaviors, such as gestures, changes in tone of voice, or the spontaneous expression of emotion" (15, p. 488). While there are different models of parenting, Maccoby and Martin (31) classified parenting style into two-dimensional framework: parental demandingness (demands, supervision, disciplinary efforts) and parental responsiveness (supportive and acquiescence to the child's needs). However, in Chinese culture, parental control is a distinctive feature of Chinese parenting (32). As suggested by Chao (9), parental control is associated with the concept of "training", which may be influenced by Confucian ideas (p. 1117). Chinese parenting based on indigenous concepts utilized behavioral control, expressed by the terms "*jiao xun*" (to train) and "*guan*" (to govern). There was empirical support that traditional Chinese socialization practices appeared to be more restrictive and controlling (2,33,34). Thus, as important aspects of parenting characteristics, it is illuminating and worthwhile to explore both parenting styles and parental control in relations to parental beliefs.

In this study, two research questions were addressed. The first question is: are there any relationships between parental beliefs (Chinese cultural beliefs about adversity, attribution of children's success and failure to effort, and expectations of children's future) and parenting styles and practices in economically disadvantaged families? The relationships of paternal beliefs and maternal beliefs with various family processes were examined separately in this study. Based on ecological-cultural perspective and the family resiliency model (12), it was hypothesized that stronger endorsement of positive Chinese cultural beliefs about adversity, stronger attribution of children's success and failure to effort, and higher expectations of children's future in fathers would be related to higher paternal endorsement of parenting styles and higher level of paternal control. Identical hypotheses were formulated for the mothers.

The second research question is: what is the relative importance of parental beliefs (Chinese cultural beliefs about adversity, attribution of children's success and failure to effort, and expectations of children's future) in predicting parenting styles and parental control of fathers and mothers experiencing economic disadvantage? As research on this area is non-existent, it is theoretically and practically interesting to explore the relative importance of paternal and maternal beliefs in predicting parenting characteristics.

METHODS

A cross-sectional survey with purposeful sampling was conducted. Fathers and mothers having at least one child aged 11 to 16 from intact Chinese families experiencing economic disadvantage were invited to participate in the study. The concept of relative poverty was adopted, with 50% of monthly median domestic household income according to Hong Kong Population By-census 2006 used as the poverty threshold. Families experiencing economic disadvantage were identified and recruited by children and youth service centers, school social work services, and community centers across Hong Kong. Finally, there were 276 families participated in the study. There was one set of invalid questionnaires, leaving 275 sets of questionnaires for analyses.

Either the first author or trained social workers conducted the data collection. Both fathers and mothers were given explanations about the purpose of the research, procedure of data collection, the rights of respondents to voluntarily participate and withdrawal from the study, as well as the use of the data in the study. Informed consent was obtained. Fathers and mothers were requested to complete the Father Questionnaire and Mother Questionnaire respectively which contained measures of Chinese cultural beliefs about adversity, expectation on children's future, causal attribution on children's success and failure to effort, parenting style and parental control. To ensure confidentiality, the questionnaire was completed by each participant separately. The questionnaire was administered in a self-administered format. In case the participants had difficulties comprehending the questionnaires, the first author or trained social workers would ask questions or items in an interview format. Parents took around 45 minutes to one hour to complete the questionnaires, depending on their literacy level.

The mean ages of the fathers and mothers were 49.94 (SD = 9.28) and 42.18 (SD = 4.97), respectively. Most fathers were born in Hong Kong (n = 98, 35.6%) or had resided in Hong Kong for more than 20 years (n = 115, 41.8%), whereas the mode of duration of stay of mothers in Hong Kong was between 6 and 10 years (n = 103, 37.5%). Regarding the educational attainment of fathers and mothers, a majority were of low educational standard, with 205 fathers (74.5%) and 204 mothers (74.2%) at the junior secondary level or lower. There were 211 (76.7%) fathers who had a job, 30 (10.9%) were unemployed, and 26 (9.5%) were retired. A high proportion of mothers were housewives (n = 199, 72.4%). The average number of children in the families was 2.34 (SD = .90). There were 96 families receiving Comprehensive Social Security Assistance from the Government, representing 34.8% of the sample.

Instruments

Assessment of parental beliefs

Chinese Beliefs about Adversity Scale (CBA). Shek (22) developed a nine-item Chinese Beliefs about Adversity Scale which attempts to measure the cultural beliefs of Chinese people about adversity. While two items (item 2 and item 5) are concerned with negative cultural beliefs about adversity, the rest assess positive cultural beliefs. For each item, the respondents are asked to rate their degree of agreement with the item on a 6-point scale. Examples of the items are "*Chi de ku zhong ku, fang wei ren shang ren*" (hardship increases stature); "*Hao chou ming sheng cheng*" (whether a life is good or bad depends on fate). CBA showed internal consistency and factorial validity in the previous study (22). Higher CBA scores indicate a higher degree of agreement with positive Chinese beliefs about adversity. Reliability analyses showed that both FCBA (fathers' responses of CBA) and MCBA (mothers' responses of CBA) had acceptable reliability in this study (α = .661 for FCBA and α = .610 for MCBA, respectively).

Parents' Attributions Questionnaire (PAQ). The scale was based on the Causal Attribution Scale Questionnaire (CASQ) developed by Chan (35), revised by Chan and Moore (36), and standardized in Hong Kong (37). The CASQ was developed within the framework of Weiner's (38,39) theory of attribution of one's success/failure and the literature on strategy attributes (35,40,41). Four attributes – effort, ability, strategy use and luck – were identified for success and failure in school children in relation with their schoolwork (36). The Parents' Attributions Questionnaire contains 24 items based on the items of the CASQ. There are 12 statements reflecting success and 12 reflecting failure. Each statement is representative of one of the four causes (effort, ability, strategy use and luck). Parents are requested to rate their agreement with each statement on a Likert scale ranging from "Strongly disagree" to "Strongly agree". Some example items are: "If my child completes a worksheet well, it is most likely because he/she is lucky"; "When my child does well in exams, it is most likely because he/she has effective strategies".

The scale showed internal consistency and factorial validity in previous study (42). In the present study, the subscale on "attribution of children's success and failure to effort" Subscale (FAQ-E for fathers' responses and MAQ-E for mothers' responses respectively) was used to indicate parental attribution of children's success and failure to effort. Reliability analyses showed that both FAQ-E and MAQ-E had acceptable reliability in this study (α = .697 for FAQ-E and α = .743 for MAQ-E, respectively).

Parental Expectations of Children's Future Scale (PECF). Based on the literature of parental expectations of children's future (43-45) and parents' attributes of an ideal child (46), as well as qualitative findings from focus groups of parents and adolescents, an indigenous scale assessing parental expectation of children's future was developed (4). The scale was developed with 23 items measuring dimensions of parental expectations on children's future in terms of educational achievement, self-reliance, occupation, family obligation and conduct. A revised PECF with 17 items was assessed in a previous validation study and both fathers' responses (FECF) and mothers' responses (MECF) of the measure showed internal consistency, divergent validity and factorial validity (47).

Participants were requested to rate the degree of agreement with each item on a 6-point Likert scale ranging from "Strongly agree" to "Strongly disagree". Examples of the items are "I expect my child to complete university"; "I hope that my child can stand out from the crowd in his/her career". Higher scores indicate higher parental expectations of children's future. Reliability analyses showed that both FECF and MECF had good reliability in this study (α = .883 for FECF and .879 for MECF, respectively).

Assessment of parenting characteristics

Paternal Parenting Style Scale (FPS) and Maternal Parenting Style Scale (MPS). Based on the framework of Maccoby and Martin (31) and parenting assessment work of Lamborn et al. (48), Shek (49) developed a modified version of the Paternal/Maternal Parenting Style Scale (FPS/MPS).

There are two subscales of this scale, including Paternal/Maternal Demandingness Scale (FDEM/MDEM) which assess demandingness of the father and mother toward the child's behaviors, and Paternal/Maternal Responsiveness Scale (FRES/MRES) assessing responsiveness of the father and mother to the child's behaviors. There are 7 items in the Demandingness Scale and 13 items in the Responsiveness Scale. The scales were found to be valid and reliable in the Chinese culture (49-51). Higher Paternal/Maternal Parenting Style Scale scores indicate more positive parenting attributes. Reliability analyses showed that both FPS and MPS had satisfactory reliability in this study (α = .807 and .701, respectively).

Chinese Paternal Control Scale (FCS) and Chinese Maternal Control Scale (MCS). Based on a review of the literature, Shek (52,53) developed a twelve-item Chinese Paternal/Maternal Control Scale to assess control based on indigenous Chinese cultural concepts. Parents were requested to rate the degree of agreement with each item on a 4-point scale ranging from "Strongly agree" to "Strongly disagree". Examples of the items are "I expect my child to be mature (*sheng xing*)"; "I expect my child to have good behavior so that he/ she will not be criticized by others as having no family teaching (*wu jiao jiao*)". The FCS and MCS showed internal consistency and divergent validity in the adolescent sample (53).

The total score of the items in each scale is an indicator of the degree of parental control based on Chinese concepts, with a higher score indicating a higher level of Chinese parental control. Reliability analyses showed that both FCS and MCS had satisfactory reliability in this study ($\alpha = .850$ and .872, respectively).

FINDINGS

To analyse the relationships between various measures of parental beliefs and parenting, Pearson correlation analyses were performed. The relationships of paternal beliefs and maternal beliefs with parenting styles and practices were examined separately. In order to decrease the chance of committing Type I error, a conservative alpha level based on Bonferroni correction (alpha = .05/6, i.e. .008) was adopted.

When assessing the correlations of demographic data with parental beliefs and parenting characteristics, it was found that paternal parenting style (FPS) was significantly associated with age of adolescents ($r = -.294$, $p < .001$), educational level of adolescents ($r = -.275$, $p < .001$) and number of children ($r = -.217$, $p < .001$), suggesting that the older the adolescents, the higher educational level of adolescents and the more the children would have relatively lower endorsement of positive parenting style of fathers. The amount of overlap on the correlation of FPS and age of adolescents, educational levels of adolescents and number of children were 8.64%, 7.56% and 4.71% of the variance. Thus, partial correlations of FPS scores by age of adolescents, educational levels of adolescents and number of children were carried out. Similarly, maternal parenting style (MPS) was significantly associated with age of adolescents ($r = -.282$, $p < .001$) and educational level of adolescents ($r = -.237$, $p < .001$), suggesting that the older and the higher educational level of adolescents would have relatively less endorsement of positive parenting style of mothers. The amount of overlap on the correlation of MPS and age of adolescents and educational level of adolescents were 8.41%, and 6.05% of the variance, so partial correlations of MPS scores by age of adolescents and educational levels of adolescents were carried out

Research question 1

From fathers' reports, it was found that fathers' endorsement of positive Chinese cultural beliefs about adversity was significantly related to fathers' endorsement of positive parenting style ($r = .238$, $p < .001$). The relationships remained significant with age, educational level of adolescents and number of children being controlled ($r = .207$, $p < .001$). However, it was found that the relationship between fathers' endorsement of Chinese cultural beliefs about adversity and paternal control was not significant ($r = .081$, $p > .008$).

It was found that fathers' attribution of children's success and failure to effort was significantly related to fathers' endorsement of positive parenting style (r = .201, p < .008). The relationships remained significant with age, educational level of adolescents and number of children being controlled (r = .202, p < .008). It was found that fathers' attribution of children's success and failure to effort was associated with higher level of paternal control (r = .303, p < .001), indicating medium effect size.

Fathers' expectations of children's future were positively related to fathers' endorsement of positive parenting style (r = .201, p < .008). The relationships remained significant with age, educational level of adolescents and number of children being controlled (r = .197, p < .008). It was found that fathers' expectations of children's future was associated with higher level of paternal control (r = .487, p < .001). The effect size was considered large. Table 1 shows the correlations of paternal beliefs and paternal parenting characteristics reported by fathers. From mothers' reports, it was found that mothers' Chinese cultural beliefs about adversity was neither correlated significantly with mothers' positive parenting style (r = .147, p > .008), nor with maternal control (r = .141, p > .008).

Table 1. Correlations of paternal beliefs and parenting characteristics reported by fathers

		Father		
		FCBA	FAQ-E	FECF
Father	FPS	.238* (.207*)[a]	.201* (.202*)[a]	.201* (.197*)[a]
	FCS	.081ns	.303*	.487*

Note 1.* p < .008 (Bonferroni correction was adopted to guard against familywise Type I error).

Note 2. [a] The number in parentheses was the correlation coefficient was calculated with age and educational level of adolescents, and number of children having controlled.

Note 3. FCBA=Chinese Beliefs about Adversity Scale completed by fathers. FAQ-E= Fathers' Attributions Questionnaire - Effort Subscale. FECF=Paternal Expectations of Children's Future Scale completed by fathers. FPS= Paternal Parenting Style Scale completed by fathers. FCS= Paternal Control Scale completed by fathers.

Table 2. Correlations of maternal beliefs and parenting characteristics reported by mothers

		Mother		
		MCBA	MAQ-E	MECF
Mother	MPS	.147ns (.133ns)[a]	.039ns (.048ns)[a]	.164* (.172*)[a]
	MCS	.141ns	.299*	.530*

Note 1.* p < .008 (Bonferroni correction was adopted to guard against familywise Type I error).

Note 2. [a] The number in parentheses was the correlation coefficient calculated with age and educational level of adolescents having controlled.

Note 3. MCBA=Chinese Beliefs about Adversity Scale completed by mothers. MAQ-E= Mothers' Attributions Questionnaire - Effort Subscale. MECF=Maternal Expectations of Children's Future Scale completed by mothers. MPS= Maternal Parenting Style Scale completed by mothers. MCS= Maternal Control Scale completed by mothers.

Similarly, mothers' attribution of children's success and failure to effort was not significantly related to mothers' positive parenting style ($r = .039$, $p > .008$). However, mothers' attribution of children's success and failure to effort was significantly correlated with maternal control with Pearson's r at .299 ($p < .001$), with a medium effect size. Furthermore, maternal expectations of children's future were positively related to maternal endorsement of parenting style, with Pearson's r at .164 ($p < .008$). With the control of age and educational level of adolescents, the relationship remained significant ($r = .172$, $p < .008$). Maternal expectations of children's future were also significantly correlated with higher level of maternal control with Pearson's r at .530, ($p < .001$), indicating a large effect size. Table 2 shows the correlations of maternal beliefs and maternal parenting characteristics reported by mothers.

Research question 2

Hierarchical regression analyses were performed to understand the relative importance of different parental beliefs on parenting characteristics of fathers and mothers experiencing economic disadvantage respectively. In fathers' sample, demographic variables (age and educational levels of adolescents, number of children), paternal beliefs (endorsement of Chinese cultural beliefs about adversity, attribution of children's success and failure to effort, expectations on children's future) were entered into hierarchical blocks.

It was found that fathers' endorsement of Chinese cultural beliefs about adversity ($\beta = .141$, $p < .05$) and attribution of children's success and failure to effort ($\beta = .124$, $p < .05$) were significant predictors of fathers' parenting style, whereas fathers' attribution of children's success and failure to effort ($\beta = .182$, $p < .01$), as well as expectations on children's future ($\beta = .454$, $p < .001$) predicted paternal control. The change of R^2 in Step 2 for parenting style and paternal control were .071 and .266 respectively, indicating that paternal beliefs had substantial influences on paternal control, but less on parenting style of fathers experiencing economic disadvantage. Table 3 and Table 4 show the results of hierarchical regression analyses of father's parenting style and paternal control in economically disadvantaged families.

In mothers' sample, demographic variables (age and educational levels of adolescents) and maternal beliefs (endorsement of Chinese cultural beliefs about adversity, attribution of children's success and failure to effort, expectations on children's future) were entered into hierarchical blocks.

It was found that maternal expectations of children's future ($\beta = .153$, $p < .05$) were significant predictors of mothers' parenting style, whereas mothers' attribution of children's success and failure to effort ($\beta = .124$, $p < .01$), as well as expectations on children's future ($\beta = .477$, $p < .001$) had strong influence on maternal control. The change of R^2 in Step 2 for parenting style and paternal control were .036 and .273 respectively, indicating that the overall studied maternal beliefs have substantial influences on maternal control, but less on parenting style of mothers experiencing economic disadvantage.

Table 5 and Table 6 show the results of hierarchical regression analyses of mother's parenting style and maternal control in economically disadvantaged families.

Table 3. Hierarchical regression analyses of paternal parenting style experiencing economic disadvantage

	Step 1 (β)	Step 2 (β)
Age of adolescents	-191	-.209*
Educational level of adolescents	-.111	-.054
No. of children	-.205***	-.205***
Fathers' Chinese cultural beliefs about adversity		.141*
Fathers' attribution of children's success and failure to effort		.124*
Fathers' expectations on children's future		.114
F	13.696***	11.333***
R^2	.132	.202
ΔR^2		.071

β = Standardized regression coefficient.
*$p < .05$, ** $p < .01$, *** $p < .001$.

Table 4. Hierarchical regression analyses of paternal control experiencing economic disadvantage

	Step 1 (β)	Step 2 (β)
Age of adolescents	.174	.164
Educational level of adolescents	-.179	-.117
No. of children	.040	.000
Fathers' Chinese cultural beliefs about adversity		-.084
Fathers' attribution of children's success and failure to effort		.182**
Fathers' expectations on children's future		.454***
F	1.067	17.141***
R^2	.012	.277
ΔR^2		.266

β = Standardized regression coefficient.
*$p < .05$, ** $p < .01$, *** $p < .001$.

Table 5. Hierarchical regression analyses of maternal parenting style experiencing economic disadvantage

	Step 1 (β)	Step 2 (β)
Age of adolescents	-.286**	-.314**
Educational level of adolescents	.004	.047
Mothers' Chinese cultural beliefs about adversity		.096
Mothers' attribution of children's success and failure to effort		-.036
Mothers' expectations on children's future		.153*
F	11.794***	7.017***
R^2	.080	.115
ΔR^2		.036

β = Standardized regression coefficient.
*$p < .05$, ** $p < .01$, *** $p < .001$.

Table 6. Hierarchical regression analyses of maternal control experiencing economic disadvantage

	Step 1 (β)	Step 2 (β)
Age of adolescents	.292**	.177
Educational level of adolescents	-.321**	-.187
Mothers' Chinese cultural beliefs about adversity		-.026
Mothers' attribution of children's success and failure to effort		.124*
Mothers' expectations on children's future		.477**
F	4.230*	23.461***
R^2	.030	.304
ΔR^2		.273

β = Standardized regression coefficient.
*$p < .05$, ** $p < .01$, *** $p < .001$.

Discussion

The present findings provide some support for the ecological-cultural framework (1) and family resilience model (12) that parental beliefs influence parenting style and practices in economically disadvantaged families. Regarding paternal beliefs and parenting characteristics reported by fathers, except for the relationship of paternal Chinese cultural beliefs about adversity and paternal control which was not significant, all other hypothesized relationships of parental beliefs (fathers' Chinese cultural beliefs about adversity, expectations of children's future, and attribution of children's success and failure to effort) and parenting characteristics (parenting style and paternal control) were significant. It was noteworthy that paternal child-specific beliefs, with fathers' expectations of children's future in particular, greatly influenced fathers' paternal control.

In the Chinese culture, traditional families were patriarchal and hierarchical, with power vested in the head of the household to maintain family harmony and proper functions. Fathers were socialized to take up the role of training and monitoring the behaviors of children, echoing the popular Chinese maxim "*yang bu jiao, fu zhi guo*" (it is the fathers' fault for only nurturing but not teaching his children). Besides, the literature showed that Chinese parenting was characterized by behavioral control, expressed by the terms '*jiao xun*' (to train) and '*guan*' (to govern), a socialization practice reflecting Confucian principles (9). With the expectation that their children can have a better future via education (19,32,54), fathers are committed to the role of training and monitoring. Hence, paternal control is prevalent in paternal parenting practices.

For relationships between maternal beliefs and parenting characteristics reported by mothers, the findings also suggested that maternal expectations of children's future greatly influenced maternal control. Mothers who had higher expectations of children's future and higher attribution of children's success and failure to effort would take up the role of guiding their children via maternal control, with the beliefs that effort and devotion to education could change their children's life trajectories. However, unlike paternal beliefs which showed significant relationships with paternal parenting style, most studied maternal beliefs did not show significant relationships with maternal parenting style, with only maternal expectations of children's future showed weak influence on parenting style. To account for the findings, it should be noted that parenting styles are related to the different concerns of fathers and mothers for their children. Collins and Russell (55) argued that father-child interaction mainly involves goals and achievements, whereas mother-child interaction mainly involves care-taking and routine family concerns. Hence, paternal beliefs about adversity as well as child-specific beliefs, being internalized by Confucian thought, affect their goal-oriented and achievement-focused interactions with their children. In contrast, as mothers are mainly responsible for caring and nurturing of the children, their parenting styles are more determined by their parenting roles and demands and less directed by their cultural beliefs. Regardless of cultural beliefs, mothers are tied to their instinctual roles and responsibilities as mothers. Nevertheless, maternal expectations of children's future reflected maternal socialization goals to prepare their children to become responsible, competent, law-abiding and self-reliant individuals. As a result, maternal expectations of children's future do affect their parenting styles.

It is noteworthy that parent's Chinese cultural beliefs about adversity were less influential to parenting characteristics when compared with child-specific parental beliefs. Theoretical accounts suggested that family beliefs on the meaning of adversity perform two main functions. Through normalizing and contextualizing adversity and distress, family members broaden their perspective to see that they can overcome difficulties and hurdles. Also, families gain a sense of coherence to define a crisis as a challenge that is manageable and somewhat meaningful (56). Thus, cultural beliefs about adversity would help to build family coherence and resilience in the family systemic level, instead of concentrating on the dyadic parent-child interaction. On the contrary, the scope of child-specific parental beliefs focuses on the dyadic parent-child interactions, which may have determining effect on parenting characteristics.

There are several theoretical and practical implications of the study. First, as studies on the relationships between parental beliefs and parenting characteristics in economic disadvantage families are minimal, the present study is a pioneering contribution to the literature. In contrast to the view that parental beliefs and attitudes had not been proven useful as a means of explaining variations in parenting (57), this study provides empirical evidence highlighting the importance of parental beliefs in shaping parenting characteristics. Second, the study underscores the importance of using indigenous concepts that fit the unique Chinese context. The concepts of Chinese cultural beliefs about adversity, parental expectations on children's future, parental attribution of children's success and failure to effort, parental control are indigenous concepts in the Chinese context where Confucian thoughts are emphasized. The findings suggest that parental control, which is the distinctive feature of Chinese parenting practices (32,53), was influenced significantly by parental expectations on children's future in economically disadvantaged families. The study demonstrates the importance of employing indigenous Chinese concepts in building Chinese family models on the influence of parental beliefs on family processes in families experiencing economic disadvantage.

Third, the role of positive parental beliefs in building positive parenting characteristics in economically disadvantaged families was identified in this study. As the "deficiency" paradigm focusing on the detrimental effects of poverty on the families was widely employed in poverty research (58-60), the role of familial factors on building family resilience was usually ignored. The present study highlights the importance of parental beliefs, especially those related to child-specific beliefs, on shaping positive parenting style and practice in the context of poverty. This helps to give us new light on helping the economically disadvantaged families and resolving the problems of intergenerational poverty.

Fourth, the findings provide important cues on family intervention in helping economic disadvantaged families. Instead of taking a residual model on providing tangible support for the families, the present findings suggest that parents do try effort in their children's development, when they have high expectations on their children's future and strong attributions of children's success and failure to effort. Thus, the findings suggest the importance of adopting a family-based intervention approach and promoting constructive and positive family beliefs in economically disadvantaged families. Family life education, hope-inducing programmes for parents, asset building projects for families, and parenting enhancement programs would be necessary.

Fifth, it was found that paternal beliefs had significant influence on paternal parenting style and paternal control. In the face of suggestions that low-income fathers are "not essential" as long as children are placed in supportive environments and have necessary resources allocated to their development (61), this study provides a counter-argument and demonstrates that fathers do value their parenting roles and development of children. However, long hours of work, low educational standard and cultural inclinations hinder paternal involvement in parenting. To help the economically disadvantaged families, the influences and roles of fathers in parenting is essential. Social workers have to reach out to engage fathers in family education programs. Men service should be expanded to cover parenting and roles of families.

Although this is the first known scientific study examining the relationships between parental beliefs and parenting characteristics of Chinese families experiencing economic disadvantage, there are several limitations of the present study. First, the limitation of purposeful sampling should be realized. As families were not randomly sampled, generalizability of the findings may be limited. Furthermore, as the findings presented in the study were based on economically disadvantaged families in Hong Kong, there is a need to assess the generalizability of the findings in different Chinese communities (e.g. mainland China) and Chinese people living in non-Chinese contexts (e.g. Chinese-Americans). Third, the cross-sectional design in this study has the inherent problem of inferring cause-and-effect relationships due to the lack of time order. Hence, a longitudinal research design is recommended for future studies. Fourth, as the assessment of parental beliefs and parenting characteristics was based on self-reported measures, it is possible that the relationship between parental beliefs and parenting characteristics is due to common method variance. Thus, it would be methodological preferable to use multiple methods in future study. Fifth, it was found that the internal consistency of Chinese Cultural Beliefs about Adversity Scale and Parental Attribution of Children's Success and Failure to Effort Subscale reported by fathers and mothers were not high (although the alpha values were acceptable). Neither was the reliability of Parenting Style Scale reported by mothers. This would increase the measurement errors. Hence, it would be desirable to further examine the psychometric properties of these scales in future.

Despite these limitations, the present findings are pioneering and stimulating in view of the paucity of research in studying the relationships between parental beliefs and parenting characteristics of Chinese families experiencing economic disadvantage. Essentially, the study is an active and constructive response to the criticism that the link between parental beliefs and parenting characteristics remains "the least often studied topic in the parental beliefs literature" (11, p. 282). Furthermore, besides promoting the psychosocial competencies in adolescents experiencing economic disadvantage as a strategy to help poor adolescents (62-65), the present findings suggest that family-based intervention is another important entry point in helping adolescents experiencing economic disadvantage.

REFERENCES

[1] Super CM, Harkness S. The developmental niche: a conceptualization at the interface of child and culture. Int J Behav Dev 1986;9:545-69.
[2] Padmawidjaja IA, Chao RK. Parental beliefs and their relation to the parental practices of immigrant Chinese Americans and European Americans. In: Russell ST, Crockett LJ, Chao RK, editors. Asian American parenting and parent–adolescent relationships. New York: Springer Sci Bus Media, 2010:37-60.
[3] McGillicuddy-De Lisi AV, Sigel IE. Parental beliefs. In: Bornstein MH, editor. Handbook of parenting, Vol. 3: Status and Social Conditions of Parenting. Mahwah, NJ: Lawrence Erlbaum, 1995:333-58.
[4] Leung JTY, Shek DTL. Expecting my child to become "Dragon": development of the Chinese Parental Expectation on Child's Future Scale. Int J Disabil Hum Dev 2011;10(3):257-65.
[5] Sigel IE, McGillicuddy-De Lisi AV. Parent beliefs are cognitions: the dynamic belief systems model. In: Bornstein BH, editor. Handbook of parenting, Vol. 2: Biology and ecology of parenting. Mahwah, NJ: Lawrence Erlbaum, 2002:485-508.
[6] Bubolz MM, Sontag MS. Human ecology theory. Boss PG, Doherty WJ, LaRossa R, Schumm WR, Steinmetz SK, editors. Sourcebook of family theories and methods: a contextual approach. New York: Plenum Press, 1993:419-48.
[7] Leung K. The roles of beliefs in Chinese culture. In: Bond MH, editor. The handbook of Chinese psychology. Hong Kong: Oxford Univ Press,1996:247-62.
[8] Shek DTL. Chinese family research: puzzles, progress, paradigms, and policy implications. J Fam Issues 2006;27(3):275-84.
[9] Chao RK. Beyond parental control and authoritarian parenting style: understanding Chinese parenting through the cultural notion of training. Child Dev 1994;65:1111-9.
[10] Burton L, Jarrett RL. In the mix, yet on the margins: the place of families in urban neighborhood and child development research. J Marriage Fam 2000;62(4):1114-35.
[11] Miller SA. Parents' beliefs about children's cognitive development. Child Dev 1988;59:259-85.
[12] McCubbin HI, Thompson EA, Thompson AI, Fromer JE. Stress, coping, and health in families: sense of coherence and resiliency. Thousand Oaks, CA: Sage, 1998.
[13] Shek DTL. Quality of life of Chinese people in a changing world. Soc Indic Res 2010;95:357-61.
[14] Shek DTL, Lam MC, Tsoi KW. Evidence-based practice in Hong Kong. In Thyer B, Kazi MAF, editors. International perspectives on evidence-based practice in social work London: Venture Press, 2004:167-81.
[15] Darling N, Steinberg L. Parenting style as context: an integrative model. Psychol Bull 1993;113(3):487-96.
[16] Shek DTL. Paternal and maternal influences on the psychological well-being of Chinese adolescents. Genet Soc Gen Psychol Monogr 1999;125(3):269-96.
[17] Benner AD, Mistry RS. Congruence of mother and teacher educational expectations and low-income youth's academic competence. J Educ Psychol 2007;99(1):140-53.
[18] Chao RK. Chinese and European American cultural models of the self reflected in mothers' childrearing beliefs. Ethos 1995;23(3):328-54.
[19] Chao RK. Chinese and European American mothers' beliefs about the role of parenting in children's school success. J Cross Cult Psychol 1996;27(4):403-23.

[20] Shek, DTL, Tang V, Lam CM, Lam MC, Tsoi KW, Tsang KM. The relationship between Chinese cultural beliefs about adversity and psychological adjustment in Chinese families with economic disadvantages. Am J Fam Ther 2003;31:427-43.

[21] Lee RPL. Social stress and coping behavior in Hong Kong. Hong Kong: Academic Press, 1985.

[22] Shek DTL. Chinese cultural beliefs about adversity: its relationship to psychological well-being, school adjustment and problem behavior in Hong Kong adolescents with and without economic disadvantage. Childhood 2004;11:63-80.

[23] Shek DTL. A longitudinal study of Chinese cultural beliefs about adversity, psychological well-being, delinquency and substance abuse in Chinese adolescents with economic disadvantage. Soc Indic Res 2005;71:385-409.

[24] Eccles JS, Wigfield A, Schiefele U. Motivation to succeed. In: Damon W, Eisenberg N, editors. Handbook of child psychology, Vol. 3: Social, emotional and personality development, 5th ed. New York: John Wiley, 1998:1017-97.

[25] Seiginer R. Parent's educational expectations and children's academic achievement: a literature review. Merrill-Palmer Q 1983;29:1-23.

[26] Brody GH, Flor DL, Gibson NM. Linking maternal efficacy beliefs, developmental goals, parenting practices, and child competence in rural single-parent African American families. Child Dev 1999;70(5):1197-208.

[27] Bugental DB, Happaney K. Parental attributions. In: Bornstein MH, editor. Handbook of parenting, Vol. 3: Being and becoming a parent. Mahwah, NJ: Lawrence Erlbaum, 2002:509-35.

[28] Georgiou SN. Parental attributions as predictors of involvement and influences on child achievement. Br J Educ Psychol 1999;69:409-29.

[29] O'Sullivan J, Howe M. Causal attributions and reading achievement: individual differences in low income families. Contemp Educ Psychol 1996;21(4):363-87.

[30] Shek DTL. The relation of parental qualities to psychological well-being, school adjustment and problem behavior in Chinese adolescents with economic disadvantage. Am J Fam Ther 2002;30:215-30.

[31] Maccoby EE, Martin JA. Socialization in the context of the family: parent-child interaction. In Mussen PH, series editor, Hetherington EM, vol. editor. Handbook of child psychology, Vol. 4: Socialization, personality, and social development. New York: Wiley, 1983:1-100.

[32] Chao RK, Tseng V. Parenting in Asians. In: Bornstein MH, editor. Handbook of parenting. Vol. 4: Social conditions and applied parenting. Mahwah, NJ: Lawrence Erlbaum, 2002:59-93.

[33] Chiu LH. Child-rearing attitudes of Chinese, Chinese-American, and Anglo-American mothers. Int J Psychol 1987;22:409-19.

[34] Lin CY, Fu V. A comparison of child-rearing practices among Chinese, immigrant Chinese, and Caucasian-American parents. Child Dev 1990;61:429-33.

[35] Chan LKS. Relationship of motivation, strategic learning and achievement in Grades 5,7 and 9. J Exp Educ 1994;62:319-42.

[36] Chan LKS, Moore PJ. Development of attributional beliefs and strategic knowledge in Years 5-9: a longitudinal analysis. Educ Psychol 2006;26(2):161-85.

[37] Mok MMC, Moore PJ, Chan LKS, Lai PY, Au WK, Lau NWJ. The development and norming of performance indicators in the social and affective domain for secondary and primary students. Paper presented at: The International Congress on School Effectiveness and Improvement, Denmark, 2002 Jan.

[38] Weiner B. Achievement motivation and attribution theory. Morristown, NJ: General Learning Press, 1974.

[39] Weiner B. An attributional theory of achievement motivation and emotion. Psychol Rev 1985;92(4):548-73.

[40] Borkowski JG, Weyhing RS, Carr M. Effects of attributional retaining on strategy-based reading comprehension in learning-disabled students. J Educ Psychol 1988;80:46-53.

[41] Chan LKS. Combined strategy and attributional training for seventh grade average and poor readers. J Res Read 1996;19:111-27.

[42] Phillipson S. Cultural variability in parent and child achievement attributions: a study in Hong Kong. Educ Psychol 2006;26(5):625-42.
[43] Davis-Kean PE. The influence of parent education and family income on child achievement: the indirect role of parental expectations and the home environment. J Fam Psychol 2005;19:698-710.
[44] Kim H, Rendon L, Valadez J. Student characteristics, school characteristics, and educational aspirations of six Asian American ethnic groups. J Multicult Couns Devel 1998;26:166-76.
[45] Spera C, Wentzel KR, Matto HC. Parental aspirations for their children's educational attainment: relations to ethnicity, parental education, children's academic performance, and parental perceptions of school climate. J Youth Adolesc 2009;38(8):1140-52.
[46] Shek DTL, Chan LK. Hong Kong Chinese parents' perceptions of the ideal child. J Psychol 1999;133(3):291-302.
[47] Leung JTY, Shek DTL. Validation of the Chinese Parental Expectation on Child's Future Scale. Int J Disabil Hum Dev 2011;10(3): 267-74.
[48] Lamborn SD, Mounts NS, Steinberg L, Dornbusch SM. Patterns of competence and adjustment among adolescents from authoritative, authoritarian, indulgent, and neglectful families. Child Dev 1991;62:1049-65.
[49] Shek DTL. Parenting characteristics and adolescent psychological well-being: a longitudinal study in a Chinese context. Genet Soc Gen Psychol Monogr 1999;125:27-44.
[50] Shek DTL. Linking between marital quality and parent-child relationships: a longitudinal study in the Chinese culture. J Fam Issues 1998;19:687-704.
[51] Shek DTL. A longitudinal study of parenting and psychosocial adjustment among Chinese adolescents experiencing economic disadvantage. Int J Adolesc Med Health 2003;15:39-49.
[52] Shek DTL. Perceived parental control processes, parent-child relational qualities, and psychological well-being in Chinese adolescents with and without economic disadvantages. J Genet Psychol 2005;166(2):171-88.
[53] Shek DTL. Perceived parental control based on indigenous Chinese parental concepts in adolescents in Hong Kong. Am J Fam Ther 2007; 35:123-37.
[54] Fuligni AJ. The Academic Achievement of adolescents from immigrant families: the roles of family background, attitudes, and behavior. Child Dev 1997;68(2):351-63.
[55] Collins WA, Russell G. Mother-child and father-child relationships in middle childhood and adolescence: a developmental analysis. Dev Rev 1991;11:99-136.
[56] Walsh F, ed. Normal family processes: growing diversity and complexity. New York: Guilford, 2003.
[57] Holden GW, Edwards IA. Parental attitudes toward child rearing: instruments, issues, and applications. Psychol Bull 1989;106:29-58.
[58] Conger RD, Conger KJ, Elder GH Jr., Lorenz FO, Simons RL, Whitbeck LB. A family process model of economic hardship and adjustment of early adolescent boys. Child Dev 1992;63:526-41.
[59] Conger RD, Conger KJ, Elder GH Jr., Lorenz FO, Simons RL, Whitbeck LB. Family economic stress and adjustment of early adolescent girls. Dev Psychol 1993;29(2):206-19.
[60] Sampson RJ, Laub JH. Urban poverty and the family context of delinquency: a new look at structure and process in a classic study. Child Dev 1994;65:523-40.
[61] Silverstein LB, Auerbach CF. Deconstructing the essential father. Am Psychol 1999;54:397-407.
[62] Shek DTL, Ma CMS. Impact of the Project P.A.T.H.S. in the junior secondary school years: objective outcome evaluation based on eight waves of longitudinal data. ScientificWorldJournal 2012, Article ID 170345, 12 pages. DOI: 10.1100/2012/170345.
[63] Shek DTL, Yu L. Longitudinal impact of the Project P.A.T.H.S. on adolescent risk behavior: what happened after five years? ScientificWorldJournal 2012, Article ID 316029, 13 pages. DOI: 10.1100/2012/316029.
[64] Shek DTL, Yu L. A review of validated youth prevention and positive youth development programs in Asia. Int J Adolesc Med Health, 2011;23(4):317-24.
[65] Sun RCF, Shek DTL. Positive youth development, life satisfaction and problem behavior among Chinese adolescents in Hong Kong: A replication. Soc Indic Res,2012;105(3):541–559.

In: Chinese Adolescent Development ISBN: 978-1-62618-622-4
Editors: Daniel TL Shek, Rachel CF Sun, Joav Merrick © 2013 Nova Science Publishers, Inc.

Chapter 4

PARENTAL BELIEFS AND FAMILY FUNCTIONING IN CHINESE FAMILIES EXPERIENCING ECONOMIC DISADVANTAGE IN HONG KONG

Janet TY Leung[1] and Daniel TL Shek*[1,2,3,4,5]
[1]Department of Applied Social Sciences,
The Hong Kong Polytechnic University, Hong Kong, PRC
[2]Centre for Innovative Programmes for Adolescents and Families,
The Hong Kong Polytechnic University, Hong Kong, PRC
[3]Kiang Wu Nursing College of Macau, Macau, PRC
[4]Department of Social Work,
East China Normal University, Shanghai, PRC
[5]Division of Adolescent Medicine, Department of Pediatrics,
Kentucky Children's Hospital, University of Kentucky College of Medicine,
Lexington, Kentucky, US

ABSTRACT

The relationships between parental beliefs (Chinese cultural beliefs about adversity, attribution of children's success and failure to effort, and expectations of children's future) and family functioning were examined in 550 Chinese parents experiencing economic disadvantage. Results showed that perceived Chinese cultural beliefs about adversity and parental expectations on children's future were positively related to family functioning in both fathers' and mothers' samples. Amongst the different predictors of perceived family functioning, paternal expectations of children's future was the most important predictor of perceived family functioning. The findings underscored the important role of the fathers in Chinese families experiencing economic disadvantage. Theoretical and practical implications of the findings are discussed.

* Correspondence: Professor Daniel TL Shek, PhD, FHKPS, BBS, JP, Chair Professor of Applied Social Sciences, Faculty of Health and Social Sciences, Department of Applied Social Sciences, The Hong Kong Polytechnic University, Room HJ407, Core H, Hunghom, Hong Kong. E-mail: daniel.shek@polyu.edu.hk

INTRODUCTION

Family serves as an elementary unit of social life. It is the unit of production, reproduction and perpetuation, protection of members from external threats, socialization and nurturing for the next generations, as well as providing affective and emotional support for family members. In the Chinese culture, family has been the basic functional unit of the society. The proper functioning of the families becomes the main driver for social harmony (1). This concept is exemplified in the popular Chinese maxim of "*jia he wan shi xing*" (harmony in the family is the basis for success in any undertaking), which truly reflects the importance of family functioning as perceived by Chinese people. There is empirical evidence that poverty impairs family functioning which further adversely affects adolescent development (2-4). Theoretically, the "family stress model" of economic hardship has become the mainstream model for studying the impacts of poverty on adolescent development via family processes. The model addresses how parental distress, marital conflicts and parenting behaviors mediate the effects of poverty on adolescent development (5,6).

With reference to the existing theories and research findings, one may ask the following questions: Can economically disadvantaged families break the vicious cycle of intergenerational poverty? What are the driving forces for families to create positive change? Do parental beliefs and cultural values shape the functioning of the families? These questions are the basic concerns of researchers and theorists in the field of family resilience. Theoretical accounts suggest that parents' beliefs and cultural values may contribute to positive family functioning in families facing adversity. According to the resiliency model of family adjustment and adaptation (7), the family may experience imbalance and disharmony when meeting with stressful situation. The family may take the challenge to adapt and improve the situation and regenerate itself through two important elements: family resources and family appraisal. In the family appraisal processes, there are five fundamental levels which may help to define the family crisis situations: schema, coherence, paradigms, situational appraisal and stressor appraisal (7). Cultural beliefs have fundamental impacts on two critical levels of family appraisal processes: the family's schema and paradigm. These processes determine how the families give meaning to stressful life events and family struggles, as well as play important roles in shaping the family's responses and strategies (8). McCubbin (7) reported that resilient poor families demonstrated high levels of warmth, affection, and emotional support. They sustained family rules and promoted family traditions, celebrations and spiritual connections. These observations echo the suggestion of Shek et al. (9) that there are two ways cultural beliefs influence individuals experiencing adversity. First, cultural beliefs may influence how adversity is defined and conceptualized. Second, cultural beliefs may shape coping resources and behaviors (9). Furthermore, Walsh (10) suggested that the influence of family beliefs on the conceptualization of meaning of adversity perform two main functions. Through normalizing and contextualizing adversity and distress, family members enlarge their perspective to see that they can overcome difficulties and hurdles. Also, families gain a sense of coherence to define a crisis as a challenge that is manageable and somewhat meaningful (10).

Furthermore, according to the ecological-cultural perspective, parenting goals are a manifestation of parental belief systems (11). The cultural meanings embedded in a particular culture shape the parental beliefs systems and parenting goals, which in turn influence the parental roles and practices (12). Thus, parental beliefs are important antecedents that infuse and guide parent's actions, which in turn may influence the family environment for adolescent development. The socialization model of children's motivation and achievement also suggests that the cultural milieu influences the socializers' (parents') beliefs, expectations and behaviors, which in turn influence the children's perceptions and expectations (13).

Although there are theoretical accounts pertinent to the relationships between parental beliefs and family functioning, it is surprising to note that research on parental beliefs and family functioning in economically disadvantaged families is almost non-existent. A PsycINFO advanced search in November 2011 for the period 1980-2011, with the search terms of "parental belief" and "family functioning", showed that there were only 99 publications. However none of these pertained to the poverty context (using the search terms of parental belief, family functioning and poverty/economic disadvantage). No publications were found in the Social Work Abstracts advanced search when a similar search was conducted in November 2011 for the period 1980-2011, using the terms of "parental belief" and "family functioning". The lack of research on parental beliefs of poor families may be due to the difficulties on theorization and conceptualization of belief systems, cultural-specificity of belief systems, and the lack of tools for measuring parental beliefs (14). Sigel and McGillicuddy-De Lisi (15) commented that "a clear conception of beliefs [for parents] and theoretical explanations of how and why beliefs are effective are lacking" and that literature on beliefs "is superficial, poorly defined, and while often in face validity, it is sorely lacking in providing information about construct and content validity" (p. 497).

Apart from the severe lack of research on studying the relationships of parental beliefs and family functioning, there are other limitations of the existing literature. First, there are problems on the conceptualization of parental beliefs. McGillicuddy-De Lisi and Sigel (16) highlighted four perspectives on the conceptualization of parental beliefs. They are attribution approaches, information-processing models, constructivist perspectives and transactional perspectives. It is noteworthy that the conceptions are not isomorphic with each other (16). However, there is very little research examining different conceptions of parental beliefs in the beliefs system.

Second, according to the ecological perspective, culture has critical influence in laying down the ideological values, norms, and institutional patterns that make up the 'blueprints' for the ecology of human development (17). It affects the socialization process, parenting strategies, interactions among family members, and social adaptation. This is of critical importance in the Chinese context as the Chinese has her unique culture under the influence of Confucianism, Taoism and Buddhism. Unfortunately, the cultural component of parental beliefs is often ignored. Leung (18) further noted "a dearth of theorizing and data on the beliefs systems of Chinese" (p. 262).

Methodologically speaking, the problems of conceptualization of parental beliefs bring forth the problems of measurement tools. There was a severe lack of psychosocial assessment tools in the Chinese culture (19,20). Indigenous measurement tools that accurately capture Chinese conceptions of parental beliefs are also rare in the literature. Besides, as many Chinese researches employed Western concepts of family functioning in their studies, cultural specificity in its conceptualization is often ignored. Burton and Jerrett (21) further commented on the "lack of attention given to cultural and contextual perspectives of family processes" (p. 1128). Shek (22) queried about the compatibility of Western theories and research findings when applied to Chinese people because Western family concepts and theories built on individualistic values that may not be compatible with the collectivistic ideology of Chinese families. Literature review showed that there are differences in the cultural norms for "healthy" family functioning between Western and Chinese societies. For example, based on a study of the attributes of "happy" families in Hong Kong, Shek and Chan (23) showed that Chinese parents and their children regarded the absence of conflict, interpersonal harmony, mutuality, connectedness, and positive parent-adolescent relationships as major attributes of happy family. Emotional expressiveness and communication were less likely to be regarded as attributes of a happy family, but they are important attributes in defining "healthy" family functioning in the Western societies (10,24,25). Again, indigenous measurement tool in assessing family functioning of Chinese families is indispensable.

The final limitation of the related research is that many researchers gathered information and responses from adolescents only (26-28), with parents' perspectives often being neglected. As each set of respondents only represents one perspective, employment of a single perspective to understand the association would confine the findings to one particular response set. On the contrary, a multiple perspective to study family processes can give us a broader scope. Day et al. (29) argued that responses from one person in family research provide a very limited basis for understanding family decisions and interactions, and thus they called for research strategies that include the collective perceptions of multiple family members. Besides, collecting data from a single data source would increase individual response bias. Even in the studies that focused on parents' perspective, the role of primary caregivers, mostly the mothers, was the main focus (30-33) with the fathers usually not covered. In short, studies including the perspectives of both fathers and mothers are rare and this limitation has hindered the building of family models in poor families.

Among the very limited literature on parental beliefs in the context of poverty, two dimensions of parental beliefs, beliefs about adversity, and child-specific beliefs, are worth noting. Cultural beliefs contribute to the belief systems of parents about adversity by influencing how adversity is defined and conceptualized, as well as by shaping coping resources and behaviors (9). Parents with strong beliefs to overcome adversity tend to act positively in the face of difficulties and challenges, which in turn influences their children's development. In Chinese communities, Lee (34) suggested that traditional beliefs help those in lower social-economic strata cope with stress from economic striving. However, he gave this a negative connotation that people use mythical explanations and manipulations of life's vicissitudes to cope with stress (34, p. 203). The mechanisms of how this explanation and manipulation buffers poor families' stress remained unexplored.

Recently, effort has been made in the conceptualization of Chinese cultural beliefs about adversity and exploration of the relationships between endorsement of positive Chinese beliefs about adversity and psychological development of adolescents (9,35,36). Shek (35) classified Chinese cultural beliefs about adversity into two categories. Positive beliefs about adversity are cultural beliefs that emphasize the positive value of adversity and people's capacity to overcome it. These cultural beliefs are basically shaped by the Confucian emphasis on people's inner strengths and virtues, such as perseverance and tolerance. On the other hand, negative beliefs about adversity are cultural beliefs that suggest impossibility and people's incapability to change adverse situations, as adversity may be due to fate or superstition. Some of these beliefs are also influenced by Buddhist and Taoist thoughts (35).

However, relationships of Chinese cultural beliefs about adversity and family functioning in Chinese families were unexplored.

Regarding child-specific parental beliefs, Eccles et al. (13) identified six child-specific parental beliefs: 1) causal attributions for children's performance; 2) perceptions of the difficulty of a specific task; 3) expectations for their children's success, and confidence in their children's abilities; 4) beliefs about the value of the specific task; 5) differential achievement standards of fulfilling the task; and 6) beliefs about the external barriers to success (13, pp. 1058-1059). Among these, parental expectation is one of the most significant factors predicting children's cognitive and psychological competence (31,37-39). This is especially important in the Chinese culture as parental expectations of children's future are deeply shaped by Confucian philosophy (14). There is a popular Chinese motto of "*wang zi cheng long*" (expecting the son to become dragon) that truly reflects the essence of parental expectations of children's future, with dragon symbolizes "supremacy" in Chinese culture.

Another parental child-specific belief that influences the development and achievement of their children is causal attributions for children's success and failure. Causal attributions directly impact parent's affective responses, parenting practices and involvement in children's activities, which in turn influences children and adolescent development (40-42). In the Chinese culture, effort in education is emphasized, as reflected by the sayings "*qin you gong, xi wu yi*" (reward lies ahead of diligence but nothing is gained by indolence), "*zhang qin bu zhou*" (diligence is a means by which one makes up for one's dullness). Thus, effort is an important parental attribution of children's success and failure according to Chinese philosophy.

Regarding family functioning, it is a complex construct which is generally regarded as "the quality of family life at the systemic level, such as wellness, competence, strengths, and weaknesses of a family" (28, p. 518). To conceptualize the construct, Walsh (10,43) identified several processes for assessing healthy family functioning: connectedness, respect for individual differences and autonomy, positive couple relationship, nurturance and care-taking of family members, organizational stability, adaptability, open communication, effective problem-solving and conflict-resolution processes, a shared belief system with mutual trust, and adequate resources for basic security and psychosocial support. With reference to the Chinese culture, Chinese parents regarded the absence of conflict, interpersonal harmony, mutuality, connectedness, and positive parent-adolescent relationships as the major attributes of a happy family. Emotional expressiveness and communication were less likely to be regarded as attributes of a happy family (23).

Two research questions were formulated in this study. The first question is: are there any relationships between parental beliefs (Chinese cultural beliefs about adversity, attribution of children's success and failure to effort, and expectations of children's future) and family functioning in economically disadvantaged families? The relationships of paternal and maternal beliefs with paternal and maternal perceptions of family functioning were examined separately in this study. Based on ecological-cultural perspective and the family resiliency model (8), it was hypothesized that paternal and maternal endorsement of positive Chinese cultural beliefs about adversity would be related to higher levels of perceived family functioning (Hypotheses 1a and 1b). Based on the ecological-cultural perspective (11) and socialization models of children's motivation and achievement (13), it was further hypothesized that paternal and maternal attributions of children's success and failure to effort would be positively related to family functioning perceived by the parents (Hypotheses 2a and 2b). Finally, paternal and maternal expectations of children's future would be associated with family functioning perceived by the fathers and mothers (Hypotheses 3a and 3b).

In addition, an overall parental perception of family functioning by aggregating the fathers' and mothers' score of measures of family functioning of each family was suggested to represent an 'integrated' parental perspective of family functioning due to three justifications. First, as each member might have some biases on perceiving the family, the employment of aggregation of both paternal and maternal scores would minimize the problems of individual response bias and reach a more integrated (though artificial in nature) picture of family functioning. Second, this practice has been used in research on family processes, such as research studying family functioning by averaging the scores of adolescents', mothers' and fathers' perceptions to get an integrated perspective (26), research studying parenting styles by aggregating and averaging fathers' and mothers' scores of perception to get an overall parental measure (44-46). Third, for further justification of the practice, it is necessary to investigate the data of each source on their correlations amongst others. If the data of different sources are significantly correlated amongst themselves, the practice of aggregation of the responses is empirically supported (26).

As research on this area is almost non-existent, it is theoretically and practically interesting to explore the relationships between paternal and maternal beliefs and "integrated" perceptions of family functioning. It was hypothesized that paternal and maternal endorsement of positive Chinese cultural beliefs about adversity, paternal and maternal attributions of children's success and failure to effort, and paternal and maternal expectations of children's future would be positively associated with the "integrated" perceptions of family functioning (Hypotheses 4a to 4f).

The second research question is: what is the relative importance of paternal and maternal beliefs (Chinese cultural beliefs about adversity, attribution of children's success and failure to effort, and expectations of children's future) in predicting family functioning in families experiencing economic disadvantage? It is argued that paternal and maternal perspectives would give us a clearer picture on the relative influences of parental beliefs on family functioning based on gender. As Chinese families are patriarchal and hierarchical, with fathers exhibited higher power to maintain harmony and proper function (47), it is essential to understand the influences of Chinese cultural beliefs and child-specific beliefs on fathers' and mothers' perceptions of family functioning separately. Similarly, the relative importance of paternal and maternal beliefs in predicting the "integrated" parental perceptions of family functioning is worthwhile to be analyzed.

Methods

A cross-sectional survey with purposeful sampling was conducted. Fathers and mothers having at least one child aged 11 to 16 from intact Chinese families experiencing economic disadvantage were invited to participate in the study. The concept of relative poverty was adopted in this study, with 50% of monthly median domestic household income according to Hong Kong Population By-census 2006 used as the poverty threshold. The economic disadvantaged families were identified and recruited by children and youth service centers, school social work services, and community centers across Hong Kong. Finally, there were

276 families participated in the study. There was one set of questionnaires that was found to be invalid, resulting in 275 sets of questionnaires for data analyses.

Either the first author or trained social workers conducted the data collection. Both fathers and mothers were given explanations about the purpose of the research, procedure of data collection, the rights of respondents to voluntarily participate and withdraw from the study, as well as the use of the data in the study. Informed consent was obtained. Fathers and mothers were requested to complete the Father Questionnaire and Mother Questionnaire respectively which contained measures of Chinese cultural beliefs about adversity, expectations of children's future, causal attribution on children's success and failure to effort, and family functioning.

To ensure confidentiality, the questionnaire was completed by each participant separately. The questionnaire was administered in a self-administered format. In case the participants had difficulties comprehending the questionnaires, the first author or trained social workers would ask questions or items in an interview format. Parents took around 45 minutes to one hour to complete the questionnaires, depending on their literacy level.

The mean ages of the fathers and mothers were 49.94 (SD = 9.28) and 42.18 (SD = 4.97), respectively. Most fathers were born in Hong Kong (n = 98, 35.6%) or had resided in Hong Kong for more than 20 years (n = 115, 41.8%), whereas the mode of duration of stay of mothers in Hong Kong was between 6 and 10 years (n = 103, 37.5%). Regarding the educational attainment of fathers and mothers, a majority were of low educational standard, with 205 fathers (74.5%) and 204 mothers (74.2%) at the junior secondary level or lower. There were 211 (76.7%) fathers who had a job, 30 (10.9%) were unemployed, and 26 (9.5%) were retired. A high proportion of mothers were housewives (n = 199, 72.4%). The average number of children in the families was 2.34 (SD = .90). There were 96 families receiving Comprehensive Social Security Assistance from the Government, constituting 34.8% of the sample.

Instruments

Assessment of parental beliefs

Chinese Beliefs about Adversity Scale (CBA). Shek (35) developed a nine-item Chinese Beliefs about Adversity Scale. The scale attempts to measure the cultural beliefs of Chinese people about adversity. While two items (item 2 and item 5) are concerned with negative cultural beliefs about adversity, the rest assess positive cultural beliefs. For each item, the respondents are asked to rate their degree of agreement with the item on a 6-point scale. Examples of the items are "*Chi de ku zhong ku, fang wei ren shang ren*" (hardship increases stature); "*Hao chou ming sheng cheng*" (whether a life is good or bad depends on fate). The CBA showed internal consistency and factorial validity in the previous study (35). Higher CBA scores indicate a higher degree of agreement with positive Chinese beliefs about adversity. Reliability analyses showed that both FCBA (fathers' responses of CBA) and MCBA (mothers' responses of CBA) had acceptable reliability in this study (α = .661 for FCBA and α = .610 for MCBA, respectively).

Parents' Attributions Questionnaire (PAQ). The scale was based on the Causal Attribution Scale Questionnaire (CASQ) developed by Chan (48), revised by Chan and Moore (49), and standardized in Hong Kong (50). The CASQ was developed within the framework of Weiner's (51,52) theory of attribution of one's success/failure and the literature on strategy attributes (48,53,54). Four attributes – effort, ability, strategy use and luck – were identified for success and failure in school children in relation with their schoolwork (49). The Parents' Attributions Questionnaire contains 24 items based on the items of the CASQ. There are 12 statements reflecting success and 12 reflecting failure. Each statement is representative of one of the four causes (effort, ability, strategy use and luck). Parents are requested to rate their agreement with each statement on a Likert scale ranging from "Strongly disagree" to "Strongly agree". Some example items are: "If my child gets good school grades, it is likely because he/she works very hard"; "If my child gets a school award, it is likely because of his/her hard work". The scale showed internal consistency and factorial validity in previous study (55). In the present study, the subscale on "attribution of children's success and failure to effort" Subscale (FAQ-E for fathers' responses and MAQ-E for mothers' responses respectively) was used to indicate parental attribution of children's success and failure to effort. Reliability analyses showed that both FAQ-E and MAQ-E had acceptable reliability in this study (α = .697 for FAQ-E and α = .743 for MAQ-E, respectively).

Parental Expectations of Children's Future Scale (PECF). Based on the literature of parental expectations of children's future (31,56,57) and parents' attributes of ideal child (58), as well as qualitative findings from focus groups of parents and adolescents, an indigenous scale assessing parental expectations of children's future was developed (14). The scale was developed with 23 items measuring dimensions of parental expectations of children's future in terms of educational achievement, self-reliance, occupation, family obligation and conduct. A revised PECF with 17 items was assessed in a previous validation study and both fathers' responses (FECF) and mothers' responses (MECF) of the measure showed internal consistency, divergent validity and factorial validity (59). Participants were requested to rate the degree of agreement with each item on a 6-point Likert scale ranging from "Strongly agree" to "Strongly disagree". Examples of the items are "I expect my child to complete university"; "I hope that my child can stand out from the crowd in his/her career". Higher scores indicate higher parental expectations of children's future. Reliability analyses showed that both FECF and MECF had good reliability in this study (α = .883 for FECF and .879 for MECF, respectively).

Assessment of family functioning

The Chinese Family Assessment Instrument (FAI). The FAI is an indigenous 33-item self-report instrument to assess family functioning in Chinese populations. The FAI has five subscales – mutuality, communication, conflict and harmony, parental concern, and parental control. Higher scores indicate higher levels of family functioning. Shek and his colleagues (27,60-62) performed a series of validity studies that examined the factor structure, reliability, concurrent, and discriminant validity of FAI and showed that the scale was a valid and reliable measure of family functioning in the Chinese community. Reliability analyses showed that both fathers' perception (FFAI) and mothers' perception (MFAI) had excellent reliability in this study (α = .943 for FFAI and .940 for MFAI, respectively).

FINDINGS

To analyse the relationships between various parental beliefs and family functioning, Pearson correlation analyses were performed. The relationships of paternal beliefs and maternal beliefs with family functioning perceived by fathers and mothers were examined separately. In order to decrease the chance of committing Type I error, a conservative alpha level based on Bonferroni correction (alpha = .05/6, i.e. .008) was adopted. When assessing the correlation of demographic data with parental beliefs and family functioning, it was found that parental beliefs and family functioning were not significantly related to parent's gender, age, educational level, occupation, family income, number of children, and sex, age and educational levels of their children under study.

Research question 1

From fathers' reports, it was found that paternal endorsement of Chinese cultural beliefs about adversity, attribution of children's success and failure to effort, and expectations of children's future were positively related to perceived family functioning, with $r = .256$ ($p <$ .001), $r = .176$ ($p < .008$), and $r = .313$ ($p < .001$), respectively. From mothers' reports, it was found that maternal beliefs about adversity and expectations of children's future were significantly related to higher level of mothers' perceived family functioning, with $r = .249$ (p $< .001$), and $r = .223$ ($p < .001$), respectively. The effect size ranged from small to medium. However, it was found that maternal attribution of children's success and failure to effort was not related to mothers' perceived family functioning ($r = .102$, $p > .008$).

Table 1. Correlations of paternal beliefs and family functioning reported by fathers and mothers

		Fathers			Mothers		
		FCBA	FAQ-E	FECF	MCBA	MAQ-E	MECF
Fathers	FFAI	.256***	.176*	.313***			
Mothers	MFAI		.		249***	.102ns	.223***
Aggregated responses of fathers and mothers	TFAI	.195*	.164*	.279*	.160*	.083ns	.127ns

Note 1.* $p < .008$ (Bonferroni correction was adopted to guard against familywise Type I error), *** $p < .001$, ns=not significant.

Note 2. FCBA=Chinese Beliefs about Adversity Scale completed by fathers. MCBA=Chinese Beliefs about Adversity Scale completed by mothers. FAQ-E=Fathers' Attributions Questionnaire - Effort Subscale reported by fathers. MAQ-E=Fathers' Attributions Questionnaire - Effort Subscale reported by mothers. FECF=Paternal Expectations of Children's Future Scale completed by fathers. MECF=Paternal Expectations of Children's Future Scale completed by mothers. FFAI=Family Assessment Inventory completed by fathers. MFAI=Family Assessment Inventory completed by mothers. TFAI=Aggregated score of Family Assessment Inventory completed by fathers and mothers.

To combine the perceptions of fathers and mothers into an "integrated" perception of family functioning, taking the aggregated data of fathers' and mothers' perceptions of family functioning was proposed in the study. It was found that the scores of responses from fathers and mothers on family functioning were correlated (r = .466, p < .001). Furthermore, result of t-test indicated that there was not any significant difference of perceived family functioning between fathers' and mothers' samples (t = .022, p > .05). The results support the practice of aggregating the responses between fathers and mothers to obtain an "integrated" perception of family functioning (26). From the "aggregated" data, it was found that paternal and maternal endorsement of Chinese cultural beliefs about adversity, paternal attribution of children's success and failure to effort, and paternal expectations of children's future were positive related with the "integrated" perceptions of family functioning, with r = .195 (p < .008), r = .160 (p < .008), r = .164 (p < .008), and r = .279 (p < .008), respectively. Table 1 presents the correlation coefficients on the relationships between paternal and maternal beliefs and perceived family functioning reported by fathers, mothers and aggregated responses, respectively.

Research question 2

Standard multiple regression analyses were performed to understand the relative importance of different parental beliefs on family functioning perceived by fathers and mothers experiencing economic disadvantage respectively. From the fathers' perspective, it was found that paternal beliefs (indexed by fathers' endorsement of Chinese cultural beliefs about adversity, expectations on children's future and attribution of children's success and failure to effort) influenced family functioning perceived by fathers (Multiple R = .364, p < .001), explaining 13.3% of the variances of family functioning. Among them, it was found that paternal endorsement of Chinese cultural beliefs about adversity (β = .175, p < .01) and expectations of children's future (β = .243, p < .001) were significant predictors of fathers' perceived family functioning. From the mothers' perspective, it was found that maternal beliefs (indexed by mothers' endorsement of Chinese cultural beliefs about adversity, expectations on children's future and attribution of children's success and failure to effort) influenced family functioning perceived by mothers (Multiple R = .296, p < .001), explaining 8.8% of the variances of family functioning. Similar to the findings based on the fathers' perspective, it was found that mothers' endorsement of Chinese cultural beliefs about adversity (β = .205, p < .01) and expectations of children's future (β = .173, p < .01) were significant predictors of mothers' perceived family functioning. It was found that parental attribution of children's success and failure was not a significant predictor of family functioning in the father and mother samples. Table 2 and Table 3 show the results of standard multiple regression analyses of family functioning in economically disadvantaged families from fathers' and mothers' perspectives respectively.

From the results of standard multiple regression analysis of aggregated data of fathers' and mothers' responses of family functioning, it was found that the overall parental beliefs (indexed by fathers' and mothers' Chinese cultural beliefs about adversity, paternal and maternal expectations of children's future, and paternal and maternal attributions of children's success and failure to effort) significantly influenced the integrated parental perception of family functioning (Multiple R = .330, p < .001), explaining 10.9% of the total variance of family functioning.

Table 2. Standard multiple regression of fathers' perceptions of family functioning by paternal beliefs

	β
Fathers' Chinese cultural beliefs about adversity	.175**
Fathers' attribution of children's success and failure to effort	.067
Fathers' expectations on children's future	.243**
Multiple R	.364***
F	13.813
R^2	.133

β = Standardized regression coefficient.
**p < .01, ***p < .001.

Table 3. Standard multiple regression of mothers' perceptions of family functioning by maternal beliefs

	β
Mothers' Chinese cultural beliefs about adversity	.205**
Mothers' attribution of children's success and failure to effort	-.017
Mothers' expectations on children's future	.173**
Multiple R	.296***
F	8.697
R^2	.088

β = Standardized regression coefficient.
**p < .01, ***p < .001.

Table 4. Standard regression analyses of parental perceptions of family functioning (indexed by integrated family functioning) in economically disadvantaged families

	β
Fathers' Chinese cultural beliefs about adversity	.107
Mothers' Chinese cultural beliefs about adversity	.102
Fathers' attribution of children's success and failure to effort	.058
Mothers' attribution of children's success and failure to effort	-.006
Fathers' expectations on children's future	.212**
Mothers' expectations on children's future	.028
Multiple R	.330***
F	5.457
R^2	.109

β = Standardized regression coefficient.
**p < .01, ***p < .001.

Among them, it was found that only paternal expectations of children's future predicted significantly on the integrated perception of family functioning (β = .212, $p < .01$). Table 4 presents the related standard multiple regression analyses.

DISCUSSION

The present findings provided support for the family resilience model (8) that parental identification with Chinese cultural beliefs about adversity influences family functioning in economically disadvantaged families from both fathers' and mothers' perspectives. According to the resiliency model of family adjustment and adaptation, Chinese cultural beliefs have fundamental influence on family's schema and paradigm, which give meanings to stressful life events and family struggles, as well as shape the family's responses and strategies (8). Parents with positive endorsement of cultural beliefs about adversity would have more strength in facing the daily challenge, and maintain a warm and supportive family environment for the family members. McCubbin (7) reported that resilient poor families demonstrated high levels of warmth, affection, and emotional support. Furthermore, families in face of adversity may experience a sense of coherence when the family struggle could be manageable with the efforts of the family members (10).

Regarding parental child specific beliefs, it was found that parental expectations of children's future significantly influenced family functioning perceived by fathers and mothers. According to the socialization model of children's motivation and achievement, cultural milieu influences the socializers' (parents') beliefs, expectations and behaviors, which in turn influence the children's perceptions and expectations. Parents with high expectations on their children would try effort to provide a supportive, affective and stable climate for their children to nurture and develop (13). This is especially important in the Chinese culture, as parents highly valued the moral sentiments of high respect for education, family obligation, and moral characters, which were rooted in Confucian thoughts (14). With the emphases of familism in the Chinese culture (63,64), parents devoted their lives and energy for the upbringing of their children. Actually, maintenance of family harmony and proper functioning are important milestones for nurturing and fostering of their children. The influence of parental expectations of children's future on family functioning is also significant for economic disadvantaged families. Parents who have high expectations on their children would create a supportive and stable nurturing environment for the development of their children in the hope that their children could be more economically competent and self-reliant in the future. This is an important path for their children to break the intergenerational cycle of poverty. However, it was found that parental attribution of children's success and failure to effort was not a predictor of family functioning perceived by both fathers and mothers. One explanation for the phenomenon is that parental attributional process is contextually sensitive, that is, it is activated to respond to an event and serves to moderate or mediate the parents' reactions towards the event (40). Family functioning, in contrast, is a less contextually sensitive process that may be comparatively stable across different situations.

As parental attribution of children's success and failure to effort is mainly related to the educational context, parents may influence their children's development via parental involvement and mobilizing family resources. Family functioning, which addresses the quality of family life at the systemic level, may not be strongly influenced by parental attributions of children's success and failure to effort.

Another highlight of the study is that paternal expectations of children's future were the only significant predictor of the "integrated" family functioning. In Chinese culture, families are patriarchal and hierarchical, with power vested in the head of the household to maintain family harmony and proper functions. Fathers, as *"yi jia zhi zhu"* (the head of the family), wielded greater decision-making power and are thus influential in family decision and proper family functioning. Being strongly influenced by familism in the Chinese culture, fathers are socialized to taking care of the family and devote themselves for the upbringing of the next generation. The findings suggest that paternal expectations of the children's future sculpt the family values which are critical for maintaining healthy family functions. The importance of patriarchal status is still salient in poor Chinese families.

There are several theoretical, practical and methodological implications of the study. First, as studies on relationships between parental beliefs and family functioning in economic disadvantage families are almost non-existent, the present study is a pioneering contribution to the literature (65). Second, the study underscores the importance on using indigenous concepts that fit the unique Chinese context. The concepts of Chinese cultural beliefs about adversity, parental expectations on children's future, parental attribution of children's success and failure to effort, and family functioning are indigenous concepts in the Chinese context where Confucian thought is stressed. The findings suggest that family functioning was influenced significantly by parental expectations on children's future and Chinese cultural beliefs about adversity in economically disadvantaged families. The study demonstrates the importance of employing indigenous Chinese concepts in building Chinese family models for the influence of parental beliefs on family processes in families experiencing economic disadvantage.

Third, the role of positive parental beliefs in enhancing family functioning in economically disadvantaged families was identified in this study. While the "deficiency" paradigm focusing on the detrimental effects of poverty on the families was widely employed in poverty research (2-4,66), the present study focuses on identifying the familial factors that build family resilience. It highlights the importance of parental beliefs, especially Chinese cultural beliefs about adversity and expectations of children's future, on enhancing family functioning in the context of poverty. This helps to give us new light on helping the economically disadvantaged families and resolving the problems of intergenerational poverty.

Fourth, the findings provide important clues on family intervention in helping economic disadvantaged families. Instead of taking a residual model on providing tangible support for the families, the research findings give us insight in the formulation of family policy that upholds positive family values and fosters effective family processes, particular for families living in poverty. Positive outlook on adversity and high expectations of children's future are important parental values that drive parents to provide a supportive environment for their children to develop healthily and positively. Thus, it is important for policymakers to promote positive family values and beliefs, as well as to formulate family-friendly policies that enhance parents to foster a harmonious, supportive and responsive family environment for their children. The findings also suggest the importance of adopting a family-based intervention approach and promoting constructive and positive family beliefs in economically disadvantaged families. Family life education, hope-inducing programmes for parents, asset building projects for families, and parenting enhancement programs would be necessary.

While it is possible to promote the psychosocial competencies of adolescents experiencing economic disadvantage via curricula-based programs such as the Project P.A.T.H.S. (67-70), the present study suggests that working with the parents and family is an equally important focus.

Fifth, it was found that paternal beliefs influenced significantly on family functioning. In the face of suggestions that low-income fathers are "not essential" as long as children are placed in supportive environments and have necessary resources allocated to their development (71), this study provides a counter-argument and demonstrates that paternal beliefs are of dominating influences on maintaining proper family functions. Paternal beliefs continue to shape the family values in the Chinese culture. However, long hours of work, low educational standard and cultural inclinations hinder the roles of fathers in maintaining a healthy family life. To help economically disadvantaged families, the influences and roles of fathers in the family are essential. Social workers have to reach out to engage fathers in family education programs. Men service should be expanded to cover parenting and roles of families.

Last but not least, there is a methodological advance on the attempt to develop an "integrated" perspective of family functioning. By aggregating the scores of responses of fathers and mothers on family functioning, an "integrated" score of responses of family functioning was obtained. The "integrated" score of responses of family functioning was assessed with its relationships between various parental beliefs. It was found that paternal expectations of children's future significantly influenced "integrated' family functioning, which showed the importance of paternal beliefs in shaping family values and maintaining family functions of economically disadvantaged families.

Although this is the first known scientific study examining the relationships between parental beliefs and family functioning of Chinese families experiencing economic disadvantage, there are several limitations of the present study. First, the limitation of purposeful sampling should be realized. As families were not randomly sampled, generalizability of the findings may be limited. Furthermore, as the findings presented in the study were based on economically disadvantaged families in Hong Kong, there is a need to assess the generalizability of the findings in different Chinese communities (e.g. mainland China) and Chinese people living in non-Chinese contexts (e.g. Chinese-Americans). Second, the cross-sectional design in this study has the inherent problem of inferring cause-and-effect relationships due to the lack of time order. Hence, a longitudinal research design is recommended for future studies. Third, as the assessment of parental beliefs and family functioning was based on self-reported measures, it is possible that the relationship between parental beliefs and family functioning is due to common method variance. Thus, it would be methodological preferable to use multiple methods in future study. Fourth, it was found that the internal consistency of Chinese Cultural Beliefs about Adversity Scale and Parental Attribution of Children's Success and Failure to Effort Subscale reported by fathers and mothers were not high (although the alpha values were acceptable). This would increase the measurement errors. Hence, it would be desirable to further examine the psychometric properties of these scales in future. Despite these limitations, the present findings are pioneering and stimulating in view of the paucity of research in studying the relationships between parental beliefs and family functioning of Chinese families experiencing economic disadvantage. Essentially, the study is an active and constructive response in exploring the link between parental beliefs and family functioning, which provides important cues for us to help the families experiencing economic disadvantage.

REFERENCES

[1] Ting KF. Meaning and practice of filial piety in Hong Kong, 2009. Accessed 2011 Nov 01. URL: http://www.cpu.gov.hk/english/documents/new/press/Filial%20Piety.pdf

[2] Abott DA, Sharma S, Verma S. The emotional environment of families experiencing chronic poverty in India. J Fam Econ Issues 2004;25(3):387-409.

[3] Berry M. Keeping families together. New York: Garland, 1994.

[4] Conger RD, Ge Xiaojia, Elder GH Jr., Lorenz FO, Simons RL. Economic stress, coercive family process, and developmental problems of adolescents. Child Dev 1994;65:541-61.

[5] Conger RD, Conger KJ. Understanding the processes through which economic hardship influences families and children. In: Crane DR, Heaton TB, editors. Handbook of families and poverty. Thousand Oaks, CA: Sage, 2008:64-81.

[6] Conger RD, Donnellan MB. An interactionist perspective on the socioeconomic context of human development. Ann Rev Psychol 2007;58:175-99.

[7] McCubbin HI, Thompson AI, McCubbin MA. Family assessment: resiliency, coping and adaptation, inventories for research and practice. Madison, Wisconsin: Univ Wisconsin Publishers, 1996.

[8] McCubbin HI, Thompson EA, Thompson AI, Fromer JE. Stress, coping, and health in families: sense of coherence and resiliency. Thousand Oaks, CA: Sage, 1998.

[9] Shek DTL, Tang V, Lam CM, Lam MC, Tsoi KW, Tsang KM. The relationship between Chinese cultural beliefs about adversity and psychological adjustment in Chinese families with economic disadvantages. Am J Fam Ther 2003;31:427-43.

[10] Walsh F, editor. Normal family processes: growing diversity and complexity. New York: Guilford, 2003.

[11] Super CM, Harkness S. The developmental niche: a conceptualization at the interface of child and culture. Int J Behav Dev 1986;9:545-69.

[12] Padmawidjaja IA, Chao RK. Parental beliefs and their relation to the parental practices of immigrant Chinese Americans and European Americans. In: Russell ST, Crockett LJ, Chao RK, editors. Asian American parenting and parent-adolescent relationships. New York: Springer Sci Bus Media, 2010:37-60.

[13] Eccles JS, Wigfield A, Schiefele U. Motivation to succeed. In: Damon W, Eisenberg N, editors. Handbook of child psychology, Vol. 3: Social, emotional and personality development, 5th ed. New York: John Wiley, 1998:1017-97.

[14] Leung JTY, Shek DTL. Expecting my child to become "Dragon" - Development of the Chinese Parental Expectation on Child's Future Scale. Int J Disabil Hum Dev 2011;10(3):257-65.

[15] Sigel IE, McGillicuddy-De Lisi AV. Parent beliefs are cognitions: the dynamic belief systems model. In: Bornstein BH, editor. Handbook of parenting, Vol. 2: Biology and ecology of parenting. Mahwah, NJ: Lawrence Erlbaum, 2002:485-508.

[16] McGillicuddy-De Lisi AV, Sigel IE. Parental beliefs. In: Bornstein MH, editor. Handbook of parenting, Vol. 3: Status and social conditions of parenting. Mahwah, NJ: Lawrence Erlbaum, 1995:333-58.

[17] Bubolz MM, Sontag MS. Human ecology theory. In: Boss PG, Doherty WJ, LaRossa R, Schumm WR, Steinmetz SK, editors. Sourcebook of family theories and methods: a contextual approach. New York: Plenum Press, 1993:419-48.

[18] Leung K. The roles of beliefs in Chinese culture. In: Bond MH, editor. The handbook of Chinese psychology. Hong Kong: Oxford Univ Press, 1996:247-62.

[19] Shek DTL. Quality of life of Chinese people in a changing world. Soc Indic Res 2010;95:357-61.

[20] Shek DTL, Lam MC, Tsoi KW. Evidence-based practice in Hong Kong. In: Thyer B, Kazi MAF, editors. International perspectives on evidence-based practice in social work. London: Venture Press, 2004:167-81.
[21] Burton L, Jarrett RL. In the mix, yet on the margins: the place of families in urban neighborhood and child development research. J Marriage Fam 2000;62(4):1114-35.
[22] Shek DTL. Chinese family research: puzzles, progress, paradigms, and policy implications. J Fam Issues 2006;27(3):275-84.
[23] Shek DTL, Chan LK. Perceptions of the happy family in a Chinese context. J Youth Stud 1998;1:178-89.
[24] Epstein NB, Ryan CE, Bishop DS, Miller IW, Keitner GI. The McMaster Model: a view of healthy family functioning. In: Walsh F, editor. Normal family processes: growing diversity and complexity. New York: Guilford, 2003:581-607.
[25] Quatman T. High functioning families: developing a prototype. Fam Ther 1997;24:143-65.
[26] Shek DTL. A longitudinal study of the relationship between family functioning and adolescent psychological well-being. J Youth Stud 1998;1(2):195-209.
[27] Shek DTL. Family functioning and psychological well-being, school adjustment, and substance abuse in Chinese adolescents: are findings based on multiple studies consistent? In: Shohov SP, editor, Advances in psychology research, Vol. 20. New York: Nova Science, 2003:163-84.
[28] Shek DTL. A longitudinal study of perceived family functioning and adolescent adjustment in Chinese adolescents with economic disadvantage. J Fam Issues 2005;26(4):518-43.
[29] Day RD, Gavazzi S, Acock A. Compelling family processes. In: Thornton A, editor. The well-being of children and families - Research and data needs. Michigan: Univ Michigan, 2001:103-26.
[30] Benner AD, Mistry RS. Congruence of mother and teacher educational expectations and low-income youth's academic competence. J Educ Psychol 2007;99(1):140-53.
[31] Davis-Kean PE. The influence of parent education and family income on child achievement: the indirect role of parental expectations and the home environment. J Fam Psychol 2005;19:698-710.
[32] Halle T, Kurtz-Costes B, Mahoney J. Family influences on school achievement in low-income African American children. J Educ Psychol 1997;89(3):538-48.
[33] Phillipson S, Phillipson SN. Academic expectations, beliefs of ability, and involvement by parents as predictors of child achievement: a cross-cultural comparison. Educ Psychol 2007;27(3):329-48.
[34] Lee RPL. Social stress and coping behavior in Hong Kong. Hong Kong: Academic Press, 1985.
[35] Shek DTL. Chinese cultural beliefs about adversity: its relationship to psychological well-being, school adjustment and problem behavior in Hong Kong adolescents with and without economic disadvantage. Childhood 2004;11:63-80.
[36] Shek DTL. A longitudinal study of Chinese cultural beliefs about adversity, psychological well-being, delinquency and substance abuse in Chinese adolescents with economic disadvantage. Soc Indic Res 2005;71:385-409.
[37] Fan X, Chen M. Parental involvement and student's achievement: a meta-analysis. Educ Psychol Rev 2001;13:1-22.
[38] Gill S, Reynolds A. Educational expectations and school achievement in urban African American children. J Sch Psychol 1999;37:403-24.
[39] Schoon I, Parson S, Sacker A. Socioeconomic adversity, educational resilience, and subsequent levels of adult adaptation. J Adolesc Res 2004;19(4):383-404.
[40] Bugental DB, Happaney K. Parental attributions. In: Bornstein MH, editor. Handbook of parenting, Vol. 3: Being and becoming a parent. Mahwah, NJ: Lawrence Erlbaum, 2002:509-35.
[41] Georgiou SN. Parental attributions as predictors of involvement and influences on child achievement. Br J Educ Psychol 1999;69:409-29.
[42] O'Sullivan J, Howe M. Causal attributions and reading achievement: individual differences in low income families. Contemp Educ Psychol 1996;21(4):363-87.
[43] Walsh F, ed. Normal family processes, 2nd ed. New York: Guilford, 1993.
[44] Lamborn SD, Mounts NS, Steinberg L, Dornbusch SM. Patterns of competence and adjustment among adolescents from authoritative, authoritarian, indulgent, and neglectful families. Child Dev 1991;62:1049-65.

[45] Steinberg L, Lamborn S, Dornbusch S, Darling N. Impact of parenting practices on adolescent achievement: authoritative parenting, school involvement, and encouragement to succeed. Child Dev 1992;63:1266-81.

[46] Stice E, Barrera M Jr. A longitudinal examination of the reciprocal relations between perceived parenting and adolescents' substance use and externalizing behaviors. Dev Psychol 1995;31:322-34.

[47] Ho DYF. Chinese patterns of socialization: a critical review. In: Bond MH, editor. The handbook of Chinese psychology. Hong Kong: Oxford Univ Press, 1986:1-37.

[48] Chan LKS. Relationship of motivation, strategic learning and achievement in Grades 5, 7 and 9. J Exp Educ 1994;62:319-42.

[49] Chan LKS, Moore PJ. Development of attributional beliefs and strategic knowledge in Years 5-9: a longitudinal analysis. Educ Psychol 2006;26(2):161-85.

[50] Mok MMC, Moore PJ, Chan LKS, Lai PY, Au WK, Lau NWJ. The development and norming of performance indicators in the social and affective domain for secondary and primary students. Presentation, International Congress on School Effectiveness and Improvement, Denmark, 2002.

[51] Weiner B. Achievement motivation and attribution theory. Morristown, NJ: General Learning Press, 1974.

[52] Weiner B. An attributional theory of achievement motivation and emotion. Psychol Rev 1985;92(4):548-73.

[53] Borkowski JG, Weyhing RS, Carr M. Effects of attributional retaining on strategy-based reading comprehension in learning-disabled students. J Educ Psychol 1988;80:46-53.

[54] Chan LKS. Combined strategy and attributional training for seventh grade average and poor readers. J Res Read 1996;19:111-27.

[55] Phillipson S. Cultural variability in parent and child achievement attributions: a study in Hong Kong. Educ Psychol 2006;26(5):625-42.

[56] Kim H, Rendon L, Valadez J. Student characteristics, school characteristics, and educational aspirations of six Asian American ethnic groups. J Multicult Couns Dev 1998;26:166-76.

[57] Spera C, Wentzel KR, Matto HC. Parental aspirations for their children's educational attainment: relations to ethnicity, parental education, children's academic performance, and parental perceptions of school climate. J Youth Adolesc 2009;38(8):1140-52.

[58] Shek DTL, Chan LK. Hong Kong Chinese parents' perceptions of the ideal child. J Psychol 1999;133(3):291-302.

[59] Leung JTY, Shek DTL. Validation of the Chinese Parental Expectation on Child's Future Scale. Int J Disabil Hum Dev 2011;10(3):267-74.

[60] Shek DTL. Assessment of family functioning Chinese adolescents: the Chinese Family Assessment Instrument. In: Singh NN, Ollen-dick T, Singh AN, editors. International perspectives on child and adolescent mental health. Amsterdam, Netherlands: Elsevier, 2002:297-316.

[61] Shek DTL, Ma CMS. The Chinese Family Assessment Instrument (C-FAI): hierarchical confirmatory factor analyses and factorial invariance. Res Soc Work Pract 2010;20:112-23.

[62] Siu AMH, Shek DTL. Psychometric properties of the Chinese Family Assessment Instrument in Chinese adolescents in Hong Kong. Adolescence 2005;40:817-30.

[63] Chan H, Lee RPL. Hong Kong families: at the crossroads of modernism and traditionalism. J Comp Fam Stud 1995;26(1):83-99.

[64] Lau SK. Society and politics in Hong Kong. Hong Kong: Chinese Univ Press, 1982.

[65] Shek DTL. Quality of life research: responses to emerging issues in a changing world. Soc Indic Res 2011;100:371-74.

[66] Sampson RJ, Laub JH. Urban poverty and the family context of delinquency: a new look at structure and process in a classic study. Child Dev 1994;65:523-40.

[67] Shek DTL, Ma CMS. Impact of the Project P.A.T.H.S. in the junior secondary school years: objective outcome evaluation based on eight waves of longitudinal data. ScientificWorldJournal 2012, Aritcle ID 170345, 12 pages. DOI: 10.1100/2012/170345.

[68] Shek DTL, Yu L. Longitudinal impact of the Project P.A.T.H.S. on adolescent risk behavior: what happened after five years? ScientificWorldJournal 2012, Aritcle ID 316029, 13 pages. DOI: 10.1100/2012/316029.

[69] Shek DTL, Ma CMS, Tang CYP. Predictors of subjective outcome evaluation findings in a positive youth development program in Hong Kong. Int J Disabil Hum Dev 2011;10(3):249-55.
[70] Shek DTL, Sun RCF, Merrick J. Training programs and implementation process of positive youth development programs. Int J Adolesc Med Health 2011;23(4):303-04.
[71] Silverstein LB, Auerbach CF. Deconstructing the essential father. Am Psychol 1999;54:397-407.

In: Chinese Adolescent Development ISBN: 978-1-62618-622-4
Editors: Daniel TL Shek, Rachel CF Sun, Joav Merrick © 2013 Nova Science Publishers, Inc.

Chapter 5

Parent-Adolescent Discrepancies in Perceived Family Functioning and Developmental Outcomes in Chinese Adolescents Experiencing Economic Disadvantage

Janet TY Leung[1] and Daniel TL Shek*[1,2,3,4,5]

[1]Department of Applied Social Sciences, The Hong Kong Polytechnic University, Hong Kong, PRC
[2]Centre for Innovative Programmes for Adolescents and Families, The Hong Kong Polytechnic University, Hong Kong, PRC
[3]Kiang Wu Nursing College of Macau, Macau, PRC
[4]Department of Social Work, East China Normal University, Shanghai, PRC
[5]Division of Adolescent Medicine, Department of Pediatrics, Kentucky Children's Hospital, University of Kentucky College of Medicine, Lexington, Kentucky, US

Abstract

The relationships between parent-adolescent discrepancies in perceptions of family functioning and adolescents' achievement motivation and psychological competence were examined in 275 Chinese intact families experiencing economic disadvantage in Hong Kong. Results indicated that parents and adolescents had different perceptions of family functioning. It was found that father-adolescent discrepancies in perceived family functioning was negatively related to adolescent achievement motivation; both father-adolescent and mother-adolescent discrepancies in perceived family functioning were negatively associated with the psychological competence in poor adolescents. The present findings provided support for the thesis that family functioning plays an

* Correspondence: Professor Daniel TL Shek, PhD, FHKPS, BBS, JP, Chair Professor of Applied Social Sciences, Faculty of Health and Social Sciences, Department of Applied Social Sciences, The Hong Kong Polytechnic University, Room HJ407, Core H, Hunghom, Hong Kong. E-mail: daniel.shek@polyu.edu.hk

important role in shaping the developmental outcomes of adolescent experiencing economic disadvantage.

INTRODUCTION

Informant discrepancies have long been regarded as "'methodological nuisances' that needed to be 'rectified' in some way" (1, p. 2). The traditional way of handling informant discrepancies was to treat them as measurement errors (2), instead of addressing them actively as a legitimate construct valuable for empirical study. Thus, very few studies have investigated the influence of parent-child discrepancies in perceived family processes on adolescent development, and research of this topic in low socioeconomic contexts is almost nonexistent. Using the search terms of "parent-child discrepancies," "family process/family functioning," and "adolescent development," an advanced search of the PsycINFO in January 2012 for the period 1980-2011 showed that there were only 17 publications. Amongst these publications, none of them was pertinent to the context of poverty (using the search terms of "parent-child discrepancies," "family process/family functioning," "adolescent development," and "poverty/economic disadvantage"). No publications were found in the Social Work Abstracts advanced search when a similar search was conducted in January 2012 for the period 1980-2011, using the search terms of "parent-child discrepancies," "family process/family functioning," and "adolescent development."

However, some researchers have argued that "informant discrepancies" are absolutely "more than measurement error" (3, p. 80) because parent-child discrepancies have important meanings and implications for the clinical assessment of children and adolescents (1,3,4). As suggested by De Los Reyes (1), informant discrepancies are important for understanding the causes and consequences of child and adolescent psychopathology and it allows treatments to be more focused and appropriate. This illustrates the need to consider parent-child discrepancies in the perceptions of family processes as "legitimate" constructs and to explore their influences on adolescent development. Particularly, it is expected that parent-child discrepancies on family processes would be heightened among families living in poverty, as expectations on appropriate parental behaviors among parents and adolescents may diverge with the availability and mobilization of family resources. The study of parent-child discrepancies in family processes may provide important clues for researchers to understand the interactions among family members as well as their influences on psychosocial development of adolescents experiencing economic disadvantage, which will shed light on how the problem of intergenerational poverty can be tackled.

Besides the negligence of parent-adolescent discrepancies in perceived family processes as legitimate constructs for empirical study, and the severe lack of research on this topic in the low socio-economic context, the literature on the relationships between different parent-child perceptions of family processes and adolescent psychosocial development is also not conclusive. Carlson et al. (5) suggested that parent-adolescent discrepancies in some domains (perceptions of role performance, affective involvement and expression, and control) were related to increased autonomy of adolescents (i.e., healthy development), but discrepancies in other domains (such as levels of cohesion and conflicts) reflected a lack of connectedness associated with poorer functioning of adolescents (e.g., self-competence and self-esteem). While there is evidence showing that higher mother-adolescent discrepancies in perceptions of decision making were related to lower levels of adolescent internalizing problems (6), there is also evidence indicating that higher parent adolescent discrepancies in perceived family processes were related to low levels of adolescent self-competence, self-esteem, emotional adjustment and social competence (7-10). In short, research findings on the influence of parent-adolescent discrepancies in perceived family processes on adolescent psychosocial development are far from clear.

Furthermore, parent-adolescent discrepancies in perceptions of family processes have rarely been studied in different Chinese contexts, despite the fact that parent-child discrepancies may be intensified among Chinese families, where expectations about appropriate parental behaviors may diverge as a function of differential orientations towards Chinese and Western cultural values (11). For instance, Chinese parents may perceive punitive parenting as acceptable based on the Chinese belief of "*bang xia chu jiao zi*" (a filial son is the result of punitive partenting behaviors), but adolescents may perceive punitive parenting as a harm to parent-child relationship, or even as an abuse. In contrast, based on the notion of human rights and humanistic values, Chinese adolescents may adopt a lower level of acceptance of punitive parenting behaviors.

Another obvious issue related to the study of Chinese family processes and adolescent psychosocial development is the conceptualization of family processes and adolescent developmental outcomes. Burton and Jerrett (12) commented on the "lack of attention given to cultural and contextual perspectives of family processes" (p. 1128). Shek (13) also queried about the compatibility of Western theories and research findings when applied to Chinese people because Western family concepts and theories built on individualistic values may not be compatible with the collectivistic ideology of Chinese families. Literature review also showed that there are differences in the cultural norms for "healthy" family functioning between Western and Chinese societies. For example, based on a study of the attributes of "happy" families in Hong Kong, Shek and Chan (14) showed that Chinese parents and their children regarded the absence of conflict, interpersonal harmony, mutuality, connectedness, and positive parent-adolescent relationships as major attributes of happy family. Emotional expressiveness and communication were less likely to be regarded as attributes of a happy family, but they are important attributes in defining "healthy" family functioning in Western family studies (15-17). Yang (18) argued that unquestioning borrowing of Western concepts and tools results in inhibition of native values, views and ways of thinking. Hence, there is an urgent need to develop indigenous Chinese conception of family processes and adolescent developmental outcomes.

Apart from the conceptual gaps on understanding the relationship between parent-child discrepancies in perceptions of family processes and adolescent development, there are also other methodological limitations in the available literature. First, some studies only employed the primary caregivers, who were mostly mothers in their studies, thus ignoring fathers in the studies (6,8). However, evidence shows that gender of the parents may also influence the relationship between adolescent-parent discrepancies in perceptions of the family and adolescent development (10). Second, the sample size was generally small in some studies: only 41 intact families were recruited in Noller and Callan's (19) study; Ohannessian et al. (10) used a sample of 74 sixth and seventh grade students and parents; Carlson et al. (5) recruited 58 sixth grade students and their parents as participants of the study. Obviously, two problems may arise with small sample sizes in such studies, including the problem of generalizability and the problem of power (20). Another common problem observed is that the effect size of parent-adolescent discrepancies in the perceptions of family processes was commonly not presented.

In summary, research on the relationship between parent-adolescent discrepancies in the perceptions of family processes and adolescent psychosocial development is severely lagging behind, inconclusive and filled with conceptual and methodological limitations. As such, there is an urge to conduct more studies of parent-child discrepancies in the perceptions of family processes in Chinese families experiencing economic disadvantage.

Among the different family processes, family functioning is an important but complex construct which is generally regarded as "the quality of family life at the systemic level, such as wellness, competence, strengths, and weaknesses of a family" (21, p. 518). In the Chinese culture, proper functioning of the families is the main driver for social harmony (22). This concept is exemplified in the popular Chinese maxim of "*jia he wan shi xing*" (harmony in the family is the basis for success in any undertaking), which truly reflects the importance of family harmony perceived by Chinese people. However, there is empirical evidence showing that parents and adolescents perceived differently on family functioning (23), with adolescents having a relatively negative view of family functioning than did their parents.

There are three theoretical accounts for parent-adolescent differences in their perceptions of family functioning. First, developmental theorists interpret the differences as an indication of individuation (24), which is a normative developmental process. The increase of family conflict between adolescents and parents may be regarded as a manifestation of the adolescent desire for autonomy, independence and identity formation (25-27). Second, parent-adolescent discrepancies may be interpreted in terms of the "generational stake" hypothesis. That is, parents have a stake in maximizing the similarities between themselves and their adolescent children, whereas adolescents have a stake in minimizing the similarities so as to display autonomy and independence (28). Parents want to nurture their children, enhance family cohesion, and provide a healthy environment for the children. Thus, they have a tendency to portray their families as positive and cohesive, as they have invested much time and effort in maintaining family functioning (25,29). In this sense, parents' perceptions of family processes may also be distorted (30). On the other hand, adolescents focus on searching for self-identity and autonomy, thus enlarging the differences involved. The differences in developmental agendas result in discrepancies in the perceptions of family processes (31). These two explanations assume that the discrepancies between parents and adolescents can be attributed to the different developmental lenses through which parents and adolescents view their family functions and interaction. In these views, different perceptions of family processes are considered normal which facilitate adolescents' healthy development (9,31).

Third, some family theorists suggest that parent-child discrepancies are the results of conflict between parents and adolescents. Olson et al. (32) suggested that the stresses within the family result in different views of family processes among family members. Minuchin (33) also suggested that parent-child discrepancies reflect family disorganization, maladaptive family interaction patterns, and a lack of cohesion. In summary, parent-child discrepancies may reveal the inability of family members to communicate and solve family problems effectively. In other words, unlike the individuation and generational-stake theses which posit parent-child discrepancies as normal and healthy, this perspective suggests that different perceptions of family processes are associated with maladjustment of families, which in turn results in poor adjustment and psychological outcomes of adolescents (8,10,31,34).

Research on parent-child discrepancies in perceived family functioning is very limited. Among the limited research, Ohannessian et al. (10) conducted a study exploring the relationship between discrepancies in adolescents' and parents' perceptions of family functioning and adolescent self-competence among a sample of 74 sixth and seventh grade students and parents. It was found that parent-adolescent discrepancies in the perceptions of family functioning were negatively related to adolescent self-competence. In the Chinese context, Shek (23) conducted a longitudinal research on the perceptions of family functioning among Chinese parents and their adolescents. The results showed that parents and adolescents perceived family functioning differently. However, his research did not further study the influences of parent-child discrepancies in perceptions of family functioning on adolescent development.

In this study, the relationship between parent-adolescent discrepancies in perceptions of family functioning and adolescent psychosocial development in Chinese families experiencing economic disadvantage was explored. Regarding family functioning, Walsh (17,35) proposed several attributes of a healthy family, including connectedness, respect for individual differences and autonomy, positive couple relationship, nurturance and care-taking of family members, organizational stability, adaptability, open communication, effective problem-solving and conflict-resolution processes, a shared belief system with mutual trust, and adequate resources for basic security and psychosocial support. With reference to the Chinese culture, Chinese parents regarded the absence of conflict, interpersonal harmony, mutuality, connectedness, and positive parent-adolescent relationships as the major attributes of a happy family. However, emotional expressiveness and communication were less likely to be regarded as attributes of a happy family (14). Thus, it is argued that an indigenous Chinese conception of family functioning should be adopted in this study.

Regarding adolescent psychosocial development, two other "non-conventional" psychosocial attributes (achievement motivation and psychological competence) were employed in the study. Achievement motivation, which is a "hope-oriented" attribute (36) that steers adolescents to succeed, is especially important for economically disadvantaged adolescents. When employing achievement motivation as an outcome to be measured, one should be conscious of the problem of cultural-specificity in its conceptualization. Most research employed Western conceptualization of achievement motivation that favors an "individualistic orientation" in determining achievement goals, incentive value of success, standard of excellence, and criteria of evaluation. Unfortunately, many scholars criticized that the "individualistic" concept of achievement motivation was unsuitable for Chinese people, which are rooted in collectivist orientation of Confucian philosophy (37,38). Hence, the conceptualization and measurement of achievement motivation should reflect a Chinese cultural orientation that emphasizes externally determined goals or standards of excellence that are socially defined and approved (38). For psychological competence, it is a composite of positive youth development attributes that include resilience, self-efficacy, sense of mastery, purpose of life, and positive future orientation (39,40). With the emphasis of the assets, abilities, and potential of adolescents (40,41), psychological competence allows a holistic view on adolescent psychological capabilities in facing poverty and adversity.

Four research questions were examined in this study. The first research question is: are there any differences in the perceptions of family functioning among fathers, mothers, and adolescents experiencing economic disadvantage? Based on the existing literature (9,10,23) and theoretical accounts of individuation process of adolescents (24), and the "generational stake" thesis (28), it was hypothesized that adolescents would perceive a lower level of family functioning than did the fathers (Hypothesis 1a) and mothers (Hypothesis 1b).

The second question is: are there any relationships between parent-adolescent discrepancies in family functioning and psychosocial development (indexed by achievement motivation and psychological competence) of economically disadvantaged adolescents? Based on the systems perspective that conflictual interactions between parents and adolescents may reflect family disorganization, maladaptive family interaction patterns, and a lack of cohesion (32,33), it was hypothesized that greater discrepancies between fathers (and mothers) and adolescents in the perceptions of family functioning respectively, would be related to lower achievement motivation of adolescents (Hypotheses 2a and 2b). Also, greater discrepancies between fathers (and mothers) and adolescents, in perceptions of family functioning respectively, would be related to lower psychological competence of adolescents (Hypotheses 2c and 2d).

The third question is: What is the relative importance of father-adolescent and mother-adolescent discrepancies in perceptions of family functioning in predicting achievement motivation and psychological competence of economically disadvantaged adolescents?

The fourth question is related to the gender of parents in the influence of parent-child discrepancies in the perceptions of family functioning on adolescent development. The fourth question is: do father-adolescent and mother-adolescent discrepancies in the perceptions of family functioning have differential influences on the achievement motivation and psychological competence of economically disadvantaged adolescents?

OUR SURVEY

A cross-sectional survey with purposeful sampling was conducted. Intact Chinese families having at least one child aged 11 to 16 experiencing economic disadvantage were invited to participate in the study. The concept of relative poverty was adopted, with 50% of monthly median domestic household income according to Hong Kong Population By-census 2006 used as the poverty threshold. Families experiencing economic disadvantage were identified and recruited by children and youth service centers, school social work services, and community centers across Hong Kong. Finally, there were 276 families participated in the study. There was one set of invalid questionnaire, leaving 275 sets of questionnaires for analyses.

Either the first author or trained social workers collected the data. Fathers, mothers, and adolescents were given explanations about the purpose of the research, procedure of data collection, the rights of respondents to voluntarily participate in and withdrawal from the study, as well as the use of the data in the study. Informed consent was obtained. Fathers and mothers were requested to complete the Father Questionnaire and Mother Questionnaire respectively which contained identical measures of family functioning, whereas adolescents were requested to complete the Adolescent Questionnaire which contained measures of family functioning, achievement motivation, and psychological competence. To ensure confidentiality, the questionnaire was completed by each participant separately. The questionnaire was administered in a self-administered format. In case the participants had difficulties comprehending the questionnaires, the first author or trained social workers would ask questions or items in an interview format. Parents took around 45 minutes to one hour to complete the questionnaires, depending on their literacy level. Adolescents took around 35 minutes to complete the questionnaires.

The mean ages of the fathers and mothers were 49.94 (*SD* = 9.28) and 42.18 (*SD* = 4.97), respectively. Most fathers were born in Hong Kong (n = 98, 35.6%) or had resided in Hong Kong for more than 20 years (n = 115, 41.8%), whereas the mode of duration of stay of mothers in Hong Kong was between 6 and 10 years (n = 103, 37.5%). Regarding the educational attainment of fathers and mothers, a majority were of low educational standard, with 205 fathers (74.5%) and 204 mothers (74.2%) with junior secondary or lower level. There were 211 (76.7%) fathers who had a job, 30 (10.9%) were unemployed, and 26 (9.5%) were retired. A high proportion of mothers were housewives (n = 199, 72.4%). The average number of children in the families was 2.34 (*SD* = .90). There were 96 families receiving Comprehensive Social Security Assistance from the government, representing 34.8% of the sample.

For the adolescent sample, there were 134 boys (48.7%) and 141 girls (51.3%) participated in the study. The ratio was close to that of the profile based on secondary schools (51.3: 48.7) in Hong Kong according to the 2006 Population By-census. The mean age of the adolescents was 13.56 (*SD* = 1.54), with the means of boys and girls at 13.40 (*SD* = 1.60) and 13.71 (*SD* = 1.47) respectively. There were 18 adolescents (6.5%) studying in Primary Five or below (Grade 5 or below), 47 (17.1%) in Primary Six (Grade 6), 63 (22.9%) in Secondary One (Grade 7), 46 (16.7%) in Secondary Two (Grade 8), 42 (15.3%) in Secondary Three (Grade 9), 28 (10.2%) in Secondary Four (Grade 10), and 29 (10.5%) in Secondary Five or above (Grade 11 or above). Regarding duration of stay in Hong Kong, 144 adolescents (52.4%) were born in Hong Kong, 74 (27.0%) had resided in Hong Kong for more than 7 years, and 24 (8.7%) adolescents had resided in Hong Kong for less than 3 years.

Instruments

The Chinese Family Assessment Instrument (FAI). The FAI is an indigenous 33-item self-report instrument to assess family functioning in Chinese populations. The FAI has five subscales – mutuality, communication, conflict and harmony, parental concern, and parental control. Higher scores indicate higher levels of family functioning. Shek and his colleagues (42-45) performed a series of validation studies that examined the factor structure, reliability, concurrent, and discriminant validity of the FAI and showed that the scale was a valid and reliable measure of family functioning for Chinese people. Reliability analyses showed that fathers' perception (FFAI), mothers' perception (MFAI), and adolescents' perception (AFAI) had excellent reliability in this study (α = .94 for FFAI, .94 for MFAI, .95 for AFAI, respectively).

Social Oriented Achievement Motivation (SOAM) Scale. Social Oriented Achievement Motivation (SOAM) Scale is a self-reported culture-specific measure of Chinese achievement tendencies developed by Yu and Yang (46). The SOAM scale contains 30 items that measures four aspects of achievement motivation: achievement value, achievement goal, achievement related behaviors, and outcome evaluation. The SOAM emphasizes goals and evaluation criteria defined by significant others, groups and society (47). Examples of SOAM scale items are "In order not to disappoint my parents, I always try to do what they expect," and "The main goal of my life is to do things that will make my parents feel proud." Responses to the item statements are reported on a 6-point Likert scale where 1 = totally disagree and 6 = totally agree. The scale has good internal consistency, test-retest reliability, convergent validity, and discriminant validity (46). The total score of the items in the scale is an indicator of the degree of social-oriented achievement motivation, with higher scores indicating higher levels. The scale was demonstrated to have good reliability in this study (α = .94).

Chinese Positive Youth Development Scale (CPYDS). Shek et al. (40) developed a 90 item Chinese Positive Youth Development Scale (CPYDS) that contains 15 aspects of positive youth development. Among the 15 aspects, 7 subscales measuring the psychosocial competence of adolescents were used in this study: 1) The Resilience Subscale (RE) is a six-item subscale that measures the capacity to adapt to changes and stressful events in healthy and adaptive ways. Some items were modelled after the items of the *Chinese Beliefs about Adversity Scale* (48). 2) The Cognitive Competence Subscale (CC) is a six-item subscale that measures cognitive skills such as problem solving and goal setting, with some items modelled after the Chinese version of the *Social Problem-solving Inventory* (49). 3) The Self-Determination Subscale (SD) is a 5-item subscale that measures the sense of autonomy, independent thinking and self-advocacy. 4) The Self-Efficacy Subscale (SE) is a 7-item subscale that measures skills for coping and mastery. 5) The Spirituality Subscale (SP) is a 7-item subscale that measures sense of purpose and meaning in life, hope, and beliefs in a higher power. The items were modelled after the *Purpose in Life Questionnaire* (50). 6) The Beliefs in the Future Subscale (BF) is a 7-item subscale that measures the ability to develop future goals and choices. 7) The Clear and Positive Identity Subscale (CPI) is a 7-item subscale that measures the development of healthy identity formation and achievement. The CPYDS showed acceptable internal consistency, criterion-related validity, construct validity and convergent validity with scores of Thriving Scale (TH), Life Satisfaction Scale (LIFE) and Perceived Academic Performance Scale (PAP) as well as discriminant validity with scores of Substance Abuse Scale (SA), Delinquency Scale (DE) and Behavioral Intention Scale (BI) (40). A Short-Form of CPYDS was developed with the items of 3, 3, 3, 3, 3, 3 and 2 for RE, CC, SD, SP, BF, CPI and SE respectively. The scale was demonstrated to have excellent reliability in this study (α = .94).

FINDINGS

To address Research Question 1, univariate analyses of variance (ANOVAs) were performed to examine the father-mother, father-adolescent, and mother-adolescent differences. Bonferroni correction was adopted to reduce the chance of committing inflated Type I error, i.e. alpha = .05/3, i.e. .017. Significant effects were further analysed by post-hoc comparisons of Tukey's HSD calculation. For effect size, partial eta-squared effect sizes are presented: 0.01 is considered a small effect, 0.06 is considered a medium effect, and 0.14 is considered a large effect (51). It was found that there was significant effect for different informants, with $F_{(2,822)} = 32.77$, $p < .001$, partial eta squared = .19 (with confidence limits from .11 to .27), which suggested the difference was in the large range (51). For parental differences, there was no significant difference between fathers' and mothers' reports. For parent-adolescent differences, it was found that there was a significant difference on perception of family functioning between fathers and adolescents, with adolescents perceiving lower family functioning than did fathers. Similar findings occurred in mother-adolescent differences where adolescents perceived significantly lower perception of family functioning than did mothers. The effect size, in terms of partial eta squared, for father-adolescent difference and mother-adolescent difference were .16 (with confidence limits from .09 to .24) and .17 (with confidence limits from .09 to .25), respectively, which suggested the differences were also large in effect (51). Hypotheses 1a and 1b were supported. Table 1 shows the means and standard deviation of measures of family functioning of each informant, and the effects of informants as well as post-hoc comparison on the measure of family functioning.

For Research Questions 2, 3 and 4, discrepancy scores between parents and adolescents in the perceptions of family functioning were determined. Generally speaking, there are three most commonly used methods to measure informant discrepancies: 1) the difference between two informants' raw or unstandardized ratings, 2) the difference between two informants' standardized ratings, and 3) the residual difference between two informants' ratings (52).

In the present study, differences between the standardized ratings of fathers and adolescents, and between those of mothers and adolescents, were employed for four reasons. First, it is the only method where the standardized discrepancy scores correlated equally with the parents' and children's scores. This allows the parents' report and children's reports to contribute equally to discrepancy scores of the variables. As explained by De Los Reyes and Kazdin (52), 'no one informant can be considered a "gold standard" by which to interpret another informant's ratings' (p. 334). Therefore, it is important that the calculated discrepancy scores correlate equally with the parents' and children's ratings so as to produce the most consistent estimates among informant discrepancies and informant characteristics (52). In contrast, the discrepancy scores computed from raw data are affected by the differential distributions of the individual scores (8). Second, the standardized approach helps to adjust the systematic biases in variability of informant responses as it empirically equates the distributions of parents' and children's ratings by the z distribution (8). This is important because children's ratings on family processes always have greater variability than do parents' ratings, resulting in higher correlation with the discrepancy scores when raw data are calculated. Third, the standardized approach enhances the interpretability of the score – the standardized score has a mean of 0 and a standard deviation of 1. Fourth, as many studies of calculated parent-child discrepancy scores employed the standardized approach (8,52,53), this maximizes comparability with related research on parent-child discrepancy and adolescent development.

In employing the standardized approach, the parents' and adolescents' reports on family functioning were converted into z-scores (the standardized scores). The discrepancy scores were calculated by subtracting the adolescents' standardized scores from the parents' standardized scores on family functioning. The positive discrepancy score shows that parents' report was more positive than the adolescents' report. Table 2 presents the correlation coefficients for measures of family functioning and their related discrepancy scores. As z-scores of the measures were calculated, it was found that the calculated discrepancy scores correlated equally with the parents' and children's ratings of family functioning.

Table 1. Effects and post-hoc comparison of different informants on the measure of family functioning

	Informant						Effect		Post-hoc comparison		
	Fathers		Mothers		Adolescents						
	M	*SD*	*M*	*SD*	*M*	*SD*	*F* value	*Partial* η^2	A (fathers vs mothers)	B (fathers vs adolescents)	C (mothers vs adolescents)
Family functioning	132.34	18.37	132.31	18.36	122.52	20.96	32.77***	.20	NS	S (F>A) *Partial* $\eta^2 = .16$	S (M>A) *Partial* $\eta^2 = .17$

*p<.05, **p<.01, ***p<.001.

Possible range of scores in the scale: AFAI, MFAI, AFAI (33 to 165 points).

Family functioning Family Assessment Inventory reported by fathers (FFAI) vs Family Assessment Inventory reported by adolescents (AFAI) vs Family Assessment Inventory reported by mothers (MFAI).

Post-hoc comparisons: *A* father-mother difference of the measure. *B* father-adolescent difference of the measure. *C* mother-adolescent difference of the measure. S significant at .05% level. *F>A* Fathers' scores higher than adolescents' scores. *M>A* Mothers' scores higher than adolescents' scores. ns = not significant.

Table 2. Correlations for family functioning scales and related discrepancy scales

	FFAI	MFAI	AFAI	DIFAFAI
Standardized scale scores				
1. Fathers' family functioning (FFAI)	1.00			
2. Mothers' family functioning (MFAI)	.47***	1.00		
3. Adolescents' family functioning (AFAI)	.35***	.39***	1.00	
Discrepancy scores [a]				
4. Family functioning perceived by fathers and adolescents (DIFAFAI)	.57***	.07ns	-.57***	1.00
5. Family functioning perceived by mothers and adolescents (DIMAFAI)	.11ns	.55***	-.55***	.58***

[a]Discrepancy scores are computed from standardized scale scores in parents' reports and adolescents' reports respectively.

*p<.05, **p<.01, ***p<.001, ns = not significant.

To analyze the relationship between parent-adolescent discrepancies in perceptions of family functioning and adolescent psychosocial development, Pearson correlation analyses were performed. Bonferroni correction was adopted to reduce the chance of committing inflated Type I error (i.e. alpha = .05/4, i.e. .013). It was found that there were no significant relationships between demographic data with parent-child discrepancies in perceptions of family functioning and adolescent development.

It was found that father-child discrepancy in family functioning was associated negatively with achievement motivation of economically disadvantaged adolescents, with Pearson's r of -.18 ($p < .013$), indicating small to medium effect size. However, it was found that mother-child discrepancy in family functioning was not correlated with achievement motivation of adolescents ($r = -.12$, $p > .013$). Thus, Hypothesis 2a was supported but Hypothesis 2b was not supported.

Table 3. Correlations between parent-child discrepancies in perceptions of family functioning and adolescent psychosocial development in economic disadvantage families

		Parent-child discrepancies on family functioning	
		DIFAFAI	DIMAFAI
Adolescents	SOAM	-.18*	-.12ns
	PYD	-.34***	-.30***

Note. * $p < .013$ (Bonferroni correction was adopted to guard against familywise Type I error).***$p < .001$, ns = not significant.

DIFAFAI = Discrepancy score on family functioning between fathers and adolescents. DIMAFAI = Discrepancy score on family functioning between mothers and adolescents. SOAM = Social Oriented Achievement Motivation Scale. PYD = Chinese Positive Youth Development Scale (with 7 subscales selected).

Table 4. Prediction of parent-child discrepancies on family functioning on achievement motivation and psychological competence of adolescents experiencing economic disadvantage

		Multiple R	Standardized Regression Coefficient (β)		R^2	*Adjusted* R^2
			Parent-child discrepancy on family functioning			
			DIFAFAI	DIMAFAI		
Adolescents	SOAM	.18	-.15*	-.04ns	.03	.02
	PYD	.34	-.25***	-.15*	.13	.12

*$p < .05$, **$p < .01$, ***$p < .001$, ns = not significant.

Note: DIFAFAI = Discrepancy score on family functioning between fathers and adolescents. DIMAFAI = Discrepancy score on family functioning between mothers and adolescents. SOAM = Social Oriented Achievement Motivation Scale. PYD = Chinese Positive Youth Development Scale (with 7 subscales selected).

It was found that father-child discrepancy in family functioning correlated negatively with psychological competence of economically disadvantaged adolescents, with Pearson's r of -.34 ($p < .001$), indicating medium effect size. Moreover, it was found that mother-child discrepancy in family functioning was correlated negatively with psychological competence of adolescents (r = -.30, p < .001). Thus, Hypotheses 2c and 2d were supported. Table 3 shows the correlation coefficients between parent-child discrepancies in family functioning and achievement motivation and psychological competence of economically disadvantaged adolescents.

To understand the overall influence of parent-child discrepancies in perceptions of family functioning on achievement motivation of adolescents, standard multiple regression analysis was performed. It was found that parent-child discrepancies in family functioning, indexed by father-child discrepancy and mother-child discrepancy in family functioning, significantly predicted the achievement motivation of economically disadvantaged adolescents (Multiple R = .18, p < .05), explaining 3.1% of the variance of adolescent achievement motivation. It should be noted that while father-child discrepancy in family functioning negatively predicted adolescent achievement motivation, with β = -.15 (p < .05), mother-adolescent discrepancy did not.

Identical procedures were performed to examine the overall influence of parent-child discrepancies in family functioning on psychological competence of adolescents. It was found that parent-child discrepancies in family functioning significantly predicted the psychological competence of economically disadvantaged adolescents (Multiple R = .36, p < .001), explaining 12.8% of the variance of adolescent psychological competence. Both father-child discrepancy and mother-child discrepancy in family functioning negatively predicted adolescent psychological competence, with β = -.25 (p < .01) and β = -.15 (p < .05) respectively. The related findings can be found in Table 4.

Correlational analyses showed that only father-child discrepancies in perceptions of family functioning were negatively related to adolescents' achievement motivation, whereas both father-child discrepancies and mother-child discrepancies in perceptions of family functioning were negatively related to adolescents' psychological competence. Thus, to address Research Question 4, only differential impact of father-adolescent and mother-adolescent discrepancies in perceptions of family functioning on adolescents' psychological competence was assessed. Z-test was performed to examine the difference between the correlation coefficients of adolescents' psychological competence by father-child discrepancies and mother-child discrepancies in perceptions of family functioning respectively (54). It was found that the difference between the correlation coefficients was not statistically significant (z = -.52, p > .05), indicating that there was no significant difference in influencing adolescents' psychological competence from father-adolescent discrepancies and mother-adolescent discrepancies in perceptions of family functioning.

Discussion

This study attempted to study the relationship between parent-adolescent discrepancies in perceived family functioning and adolescent psychosocial development in Chinese families experiencing economic disadvantage. There are several unique features in the study. First, parent-adolescent discrepancy in perceived family functioning was regarded as a "legitimate" measurement construct and its relationship to adolescent psychosocial development was explored. Second, members of Chinese families experiencing economic disadvantage were recruited as participants of the study, with both cultural and socio-economic contexts unique in the related studies. Third, achievement motivation and psychological competence, which are positive youth developmental attributes that emphasize adolescent potential and capabilities in face of poverty and adversity, were employed as outcome measures in this study. Fourth, fathers, mothers and adolescents were recruited in the study. Fifth, indigenous Chinese conceptions of family functioning and achievement motivation were adopted. Sixth, indigenous Chinese assessment tools of family functioning, achievement motivation, and psychological competence were used in the study. Last but not least, differential impacts of father-adolescent and mother-adolescent discrepancies in perceptions of family functioning on the psychological competence of economically disadvantaged adolescents were studied.

The findings support the previous research that parents and adolescents had different perceptions of family functioning, with adolescents showing lower levels of family functioning than did their parents (9,10,23). Furthermore, echoing the literature that parent-child discrepancies in perceptions of family processes were related to low levels of adolescent psychosocial development (5,8,10), the findings revealed that higher parent-adolescent discrepancies in family functioning was generally related to lower achievement motivation and psychological competence in economically disadvantaged adolescents. The findings sound an alarm that parent-adolescent discrepancies in family functioning may go beyond the normal developmental assumptions of the individuation process (24) and the "generational stake" thesis (28), which are regarded as healthy. The strength and directions of correlation coefficients on the relationships between parent-adolescent discrepancies in perceived family functioning and adolescent psychosocial development suggest that there may be conflicting interactions between parents and adolescents in poor families that bring stress and maladjustment, which in turn result in poor psychological adjustment of adolescents. This interpretation is in line with the clinical literature that discrepancies between family members in perceptions of family functioning were related to both maladjustment in individual and to the family (32,55). Parent-adolescent discrepancies in perceptions of family functioning may also be seen as poor communication between parents and adolescents, which may result in a lack of harmony and cohesion in the family (33).

In the Chinese culture, parent-adolescent discrepancies in perceived family functioning may bring additional hurdles to adolescent psychological development. With the emphases of familism as well as interdependent relations among family members (56,57), adolescents develop the concept of self in the linkage of attachment and relationships with others, especially the significant others (58,59). Miscommunication or the threat of detrimental family relationships would have adverse effects on adolescent emotional adjustment and development of self-identity. This helps to explain the negative influence of parent-child discrepancies in family functioning on the psychological development of adolescents, though further research on this area is needed.

It is noteworthy that father-adolescent discrepancies in the perceptions of family functioning have adverse influence on both achievement motivation and psychological competence of adolescents, whereas mother-adolescent discrepancies in the perceptions of family functioning have only adverse influence on adolescent psychological competence. In the Chinese culture, families are patriarchal and hierarchical, with power vested in the head of the household to maintain family harmony and proper functions. Fathers, as *"yi jia zhi zhu"* (the head of the family), wield great decision-making power and are thus influential in family decision and proper family functioning. Adolescents may perceive paternal decisions as determinative and conclusive, and thus any disagreement on the decisions may result in conflictual interactions between fathers and adolescents, which in turn would influence adolescents' psychosocial development. Particularly, Collins and Russell (60) found that father-child interaction mainly involves goals and achievements, whereas mother-child interaction mainly involves care-taking and routine family concerns. Thus, father-adolescent discrepancies in perceived family functioning would adversely influence achievement motivation of adolescents, which is more directed to goal accomplishment and success, but mother-adolescent discrepancies in perceptions of family functioning do not. Still, both father-adolescent discrepancies and mother-adolescent discrepancies in the perceptions of family functioning may imply conflicting communications between parents and adolescents, which result in poor psychological competence of adolescents.

There are several theoretical implications of the study. First, in view of the severe lack of research on the relationship between parent-child discrepancies in perceived family functioning and adolescent psychosocial development in Chinese families experiencing economic disadvantage, the present study is an important addition to the literature. Second, the study sheds new light on our understanding of familial influences of adolescent psychosocial development in the context of poverty. Regarding how poverty influences adolescent development via family processes, the "family stress" model which emphasizes the mediation pathways of parental distress and poor parenting behaviors (61,62) is dominant in the academic arena. These findings give us an alternate perspective that parent-child discrepancies in perceptions of family functioning are significant and they negatively impact on adolescent developmental outcomes. This brings important theoretical implications for studying the impacts of poverty on family processes and adolescent development. Third, the findings support the view that "informant discrepancies" are absolutely "more than measurement error" (3, p. 80) which have important meanings and implications on understanding the antecedents and consequences of children's and adolescents' behaviors (1,3,4). Hence, parent-child discrepancies in family processes should be treated as a legitimate construct that deserves academic and empirical attention.

The study also has several practical implications. First, consistent with the previous research (9,10,23) that parents and adolescents may have different perception of family functioning, it is important to take into account of different family members in clinical assessment and treatment. Second, research findings indicated that there were significant parent-child discrepancies in the perceptions of family functioning, and the discrepancies negatively influence achievement motivation and psychological competence of adolescents experiencing economic disadvantage. The parent-adolescent discrepancies may be interpreted as problems in communication between parents and adolescents that result in parent-child conflict (31,32) in economic disadvantaged families. As suggested by De Los Reyes (1), informant discrepancies can be important in both understanding the causes and consequences of child and adolescent psychopathology, and allowing treatments to be more focused and appropriate. As a result, social workers should be sensitive to differences in the interpretations of family processes between parents and adolescents, as well as the meanings of the discrepancies. Also, social workers should pay more attention to the facilitation of parent-child communication and resolving parent-child conflicts in helping adolescents and families experiencing economically disadvantage.

Third, the findings call for anti-poverty policies, programmes, and intervention strategies to be family-based. To resolve the threat of intergenerational poverty, taking a residual model on providing tangible support for the families is clearly not enough. The present findings provide some pointer for the formulation of family policies and programmes that can promote parent-child interactions and mutual understanding for the purpose to reduce the psychosocial maladjustment of adolescents. Family life education, asset-building projects for families, parenting enhancement programs, would be necessary.

Last but not least, it was identified that father-adolescent discrepancies in perceived family functioning has significant negative impacts on the achievement motivation and psychological competence of adolescents. The findings alert social workers and clinical practitioners to the fact that father-child conflict could be detrimental to adolescent well-being. As men are less likely to seek help, social workers and clinical practitioners should be sensitive to father-child conflict and make more room for father-child communication and mutual understanding.

Although this is the first known scientific study examining the relationships between parent-adolescent discrepancies in family functioning and adolescent psychosocial development of Chinese families experiencing economic disadvantage, there are several limitations of the present study. First, the limitation of purposeful sampling should be recognized. As the participated families recruited were not randomly sampled, generalizability of the findings may be limited. Second, the cross-sectional design in this study has the inherent problem in inferring cause-and-effect relationships due to time order. Hence, a longitudinal research design is recommended in future studies. Third, as the assessments of family functioning and adolescent psychosocial development were based on the self-reported questionnaires, the findings may only represent the perceptions of the "insiders." It would be more illuminating to include observation data in real-life settings from the "outsiders" view so that a more comprehensive picture of family processes and adolescent psychosocial competence can be obtained. Fourth, as the findings presented in the study were based on economically disadvantaged families in Hong Kong, there is a need to assess the generalizability of the findings in different Chinese communities (e.g. mainland China) and Chinese people living in non-Chinese contexts (e.g. Chinese-Americans).

Despite these limitations, the present findings are pioneering and stimulating in view of the paucity of research in studying the relationships between parent-adolescent discrepancies in perceptions of family functioning and adolescent psychosocial development of Chinese families experiencing economic disadvantage. Essentially, the study is an active and constructive response to the quest of De Los Reyes (1) on taking parent-child discrepancies in perceptions of family functioning as a "legitimate" construct and exploring their links with adolescent achievement motivation and psychological competence, which provides important clues for us to help the families experiencing economic disadvantage.

REFERENCES

[1] De Los Reyes A. More than measurement error: discovering meaning behind informant discrepancies in clinical assessments of children and adolescents. J Clin Child Adolesc Psychol 2011;40(1):1-9.

[2] McGuire WJ. Suspiciousness of experimenter's intent. In: Rosenthal R, Rosnow RL, editors. Artifact in behavioral research. New York: Academic Press, 1969:13-57.

[3] Achenbach TM. Commentary: Definitely more than measurement error: but how should we understand and deal with informant discrepancies? J Clin Child Adolesc Psychol 2011;40(1):80-6.

[4] Achenbach TM, McConaughy SH, Howell CT. Child/adolescent behavioral and emotional problems: implications of cross-informant correlations for situational specificity. Psychol Bull 1987;101:213-32.

[5] Carlson CI, Cooper CR, Spradling VY. Developmental implications of shared versus distinct perceptions of the family in early adolescence. In: Paikoff RL, editor. New directions for child development: shared views in the family during adolescence Vol. 51. San Francisco: Jossey-Bass, 1991:13-32.
[6] Holmbeck GN, O'Donnell K. Discrepancies between perceptions of decision making and behavioral autonomy. New Dir Child Dev 1991;51:51-69.
[7] Gaylord KK, Kitzmann KM, Coleman JK. Parents' and children's perceptions of parental behavior: associations with children's psychosocial adjustment in the classroom. Parent Sci Pract 2003;3:23-47.
[8] Guion K, Mrug S, Windle M. Predictive value of informant discrepancies in reports of parenting: relations to early adolescents' adjustment. J Abnorm Child Psychol 2009;37:17-30.
[9] Ohannessian CM, Lerner RM, Lerner JV, von Eye A. Discrepancies in adolescents' and parents' perceptions of family functioning and adolescent emotional adjustment. J Early Adolesc 1995;15(4):490-516.
[10] Ohannessian CM, Lerner RM, Lerner JV, von Eye A. Adolescent-parent discrepancies in perceptions of family functioning and early adolescent self-competence. Int J Behav Dev 2000;24(3):362-72.
[11] Fung JJ, Lau AS. Factors associated with parent-child (dis)agreement on child behavior and parenting problems in Chinese immigrant families. J Clin Child Adolesc Psychol 2010;39(3):314-27.
[12] Burton L, Jarrett RL. In the mix, yet on the margins: the place of families in urban neighborhood and child development research. J Marriage Fam 2000;62(4):1114-35.
[13] Shek DTL. Chinese family research: puzzles, progress, paradigms, and policy implications. J Fam Issues 2006;27(3):275-84.
[14] Shek DTL, Chan LK. Perceptions of the happy family in a Chinese context. J Youth Stud 1998;1: 178-89.
[15] Epstein NB, Ryan CE, Bishop DS, Miller IW, Keitner GI. The McMaster Model: a view of healthy family functioning. In: Walsh F, editor. Normal family processes: growing diversity and complexity. New York: Guilford, 2003:581-607.
[16] Quatman T. High functioning families: Developing a prototype. Fam Ther 1997;24:143-65.
[17] Walsh F, ed. Normal family processes: Growing diversity and complexity. New York: Guilford, 2003.
[18] Yang KS. Towards an indigenous Chinese psychology: a selective review of methodological, theoretical, and empirical accomplishments. Chin J Psychol 1999;41(2):181-211.
[19] Noller P, Callan VJ. Understanding parent-child interactions: perceptions of family members and outsiders. Dev Psychol 1988;24:707-14.
[20] Kraemer HC, Thiemann S. How many subjects? Statistical power analysis in research. Newbury Park: Sage, 1987.
[21] Shek DTL. A longitudinal study of perceived family functioning and adolescent adjustment in Chinese adolescents with economic disadvantage. J Fam Issues 2005;26(4):518-43.
[22] Ting KF. Meaning and practice of filial piety in Hong Kong. Accessed 2011 Nov 25. URL: http://www.cpu.gov.hk/english/documents/new/press/Filial%20Piety.pdf.
[23] Shek DTL. Perception of family functioning among Chinese parents and their adolescent children. Am J Fam Ther 1999;27:304-14.
[24] Grotevant HD, Cooper CR. Individuation in family relationships: a perspective on individual differences in the development of identity and role-taking skills in adolescence. Hum Dev 1986;29: 82-100.
[25] Lerner RM, Spanier GB. Adolescent development: a life-span perspective. New York: McGraw-Hill, 1980.
[26] Montemayor R, Flannery DJ. Parent-adolescent relations in middle and late adolescence. In: Lerner RM, Petersen AC, Brooks-Gunn J, editors. Encyclopedia of adolescence. New York: Garland, 1991: 729-34.
[27] Steinberg LD. Parent-adolescent relations. In: Lerner RM, Petersen AC, Brooks-Gunn J, editors. Encyclopedia of adolescence. New York: Garland, 1991:724-28.
[28] Bengtson VL, Kuypers JA. Generational differences and the developmental stake. Aging Hum Dev 1971;2:249-60.

[29] Lerner RM, Knapp JR. Actual and perceived intra-familial attitudes of late adolescents and their parents. J Youth Adolesc 1975;4:17-36.

[30] Niemi RG. How family members perceive each other: political and social attitudes in two generations. New Haven, CT: Yale Univ Press, 1974.

[31] Welsh DP, Galliher RV, Powers SI. Divergent realities and perceived inequalities: adolescents', mothers', and observers' perception of family interactions and adolescent psychological functioning. J Adolesc Res 1998;13:377-402.

[32] Olson DH, McCubbin HI, Larsen AS, Muxen MJ, Wilson MA. Families: what makes them work. Thousand Oaks, CA: Sage, 1983.

[33] Minuchin P. Families and individual development: provocations from the field of family therapy. Child Dev 1985;56:289-302.

[34] Feinberg ME, Howe GW, Reiss D, Hetherington EM. Relationship between perceptual differences of parenting and adolescent antisocial behavior and depressive symptoms. J Fam Psychol 2000;14: 531-55.

[35] Walsh F. ed. Normal family processes, 2nd ed. New York: Guilford, 1993.

[36] Feather NT. The relationship of expectation of success to need achievement and test anxiety. J Pers Soc Psychol 1965;1:118-26.

[37] de Vos GA. Socialization for achievement: essays on the cultural psychology of the Japanese. Berkeley: Univ California Press, 1973.

[38] Yang KS, Yu AB. Social-oriented and individual-oriented achievement motivation: conceptualization and measurement. Paper presented at the symposium on Chinese personality and social psychology. 24th International Congress of Psychology, Sydney, 1988.

[39] Catalano RF, Berglund ML, Ryan JAM, Lonczak HS, Hawkins JD. Positive youth development in the United States: Research findings on evaluation of positive youth development programs. Prev Treatment [serial on the internet]. Accessed 2012 Jan 16. URL: http://www.journals.apa.org/prevention/ volume5/pre0050015a.html

[40] Shek DTL, Siu AMH, Lee TY. The Chinese Positive Youth Development Scale: A validation study. Res Soc Work Pract 2007;17:380-91.

[41] Damon W. What is positive youth development? Ann Am Acad Pol Soc Sci 2004;591:13-24.

[42] Shek DTL. Assessment of family functioning Chinese adolescents: the Chinese Family Assessment Instrument. In: Singh NN, Ollen-dick T, Singh AN, editors. International perspectives on child and adolescent Mental Health. Amsterdam, Netherlands: Elsevier, 2002:297-316.

[43] Shek DTL. Family functioning and psychological well-being, school adjustment, and substance abuse in Chinese adolescents: Are findings based on multiple studies consistent? In Shohov SP, editor. Advances in psychology research, Vol. 20. New York: Nova Science Publishers, 2003:163-84.

[44] Shek DTL, Ma CMS. The Chinese Family Assessment Instrument (C-FAI): hierarchical confirmatory factor analyses and factorial invariance. Res Soc Work Pract 2010;20:112-23.

[45] Siu AMH, Shek DTL. Psychometric properties of the Chinese Family Assessment Instrument in Chinese adolescents in Hong Kong. Adolescence 2005;40:817-30.

[46] Yu AB, Yang KS. Social-oriented and individual-oriented achievement motivation: a conceptual and empirical analysis. Bulletin of the Institute of Ethnology, Academia Sinica (Taiwan) 1989;64:51-98.[Chinese]

[47] Yu AB. Ultimate life concerns, self, and Chinese achievement motivation. In: Bond MH, editor. The handbook of Chinese psychology. Hong Kong: Oxford Univ Press, 1996:227-46.

[48] Shek DTL. Chinese cultural beliefs about adversity: its relationship to psychological well-being, school adjustment and problem behavior in Hong Kong adolescents with and without economic disadvantage. Childhood 2004;11:63-80.

[49] Siu AMH, Shek DTL. The Chinese version of the Social Problem-solving Inventory: some initial results on reliability and validity. J Clin Psychol 2005;61:347-60.

[50] Shek DTL. Meaning in life and psychological well-being: an empirical study using the Chinese version of the Purpose in Life Questionnaire. J Genet Psychol 1992;153:185-200.

[51] Stevens JP. Applied multivariate statistics for the social sciences. Mahwah, New Jersey: Lawrence Erlbaum Associates, 2002.

[52] De Los Reyes A, Kazdin AE. Measuring informant discrepancies in clinical child research. Psychol Assess 2004;16:330-4.

[53] Ferdinand RF, van der Ende J, Verhulist FC. Parent-adolescent disagreement regarding psychopathology in adolescents from the general population as a risk factor for adverse outcome. J Abnorm Psychol 2004;113:198-206.

[54] Tabachnick BG, Fidell LS. Using Multivariate Statistics. Boston: Pearson Education, 2007.

[55] Reiss D. The family's construction of reality. Cambridge, M.A: Harvard Univ Press, 1981.

[56] Chan H, Lee RPL. Hong Kong families: at the crossroads of modernism and traditionalism. J Comp Fam Stud 1995;26(1):83-99.

[57] Lau SK. Society and politics in Hong Kong. Hong Kong: Chinese Univ Press, 1982.

[58] de Vos G.A. Confucian family socialization: the religion, morality, and aesthetics of propriety. In Slote WH, de Vos GA, editors. Confucianism and the Family. New York: State Univ New York Press, 1998:329-80.

[59] Ho DYF. Selfhood and identity in Confucianism, Taoism, Buddhism, and Hinduism: contrasts with the West. J Theory Soc Behav 1995;25(2):115-39.

[60] Collins WA, Russell G. Mother-child and father-child relationships in middle childhood and adolescence: a developmental analysis. Dev Rev 1991;11:99-136.

[61] Conger RD, Conger KJ. Understanding the processes through which economic hardship influences families and children. In: Crane DR, Heaton TB, editors. Handbook of families and poverty. Los Angeles: Sage, 2008:64-81.

[62] Conger RD, Donnellan MB. An interactionist perspective on the socioeconomic context of human development. Ann Rev Psychol 2007;58:175-199.

In: Chinese Adolescent Development ISBN: 978-1-62618-622-4
Editors: Daniel TL Shek, Rachel CF Sun, Joav Merrick © 2013 Nova Science Publishers, Inc.

Chapter 6

ASSESSMENT OF NON-CONFLICT RELATED MARITAL QUALITY FROM THE PERSPECTIVE OF CHINESE ADOLESCENTS

***Hung-Kit Fok*[1] *and Daniel TL Shek*[1,2,3,4,5*]**

[1]Department of Applied Social Sciences, The Hong Kong Polytechnic University, Hong Kong, PRChina
[2]Public Policy Research Institute, The Hong Kong Polytechnic University, Hong Kong, PRChina
[3]Kiang Wu Nursing College of Macau, Macau, PRChina
[4]Department of Social Work, East China Normal University, PRChina
[5]Division of Adolescent Medicine, Department of Pediatrics, Kentucky Children's Hospital, University of Kentucky College of Medicine, Lexington, Kentucky, US

ABSTRACT

An indigenous Chinese measure of non-conflict related marital quality attributes from the perspective of adolescent children was developed. Based on a comprehensive literature review and focus group interviews of social workers and adolescents, 14 categories of themes (i.e., respect, appreciation, responsibility, trust, body touch, togetherness, intimacy, communication, acceptance, concern, criticism, consistency, helping, and response) were identified, and a scale assessing adolescent perception of inter-parental non-conflict related attributes was developed. A panel of experts was formed to determine the relevance, clarity and representativeness of the developed items to assess the content vadlity of the measure, after which the views of the experts were used to further refine the scale. The findings showed that the final 60-item measure had high relevance, clarity and representativeness of the construct of non-conflict related

---

* Corresponding author: Professor Daniel TL Shek, PhD, FHKPS, BBS, JP, Chair Professor of Applied Social Sciences, Faculty of Health and Social Sciences, Department of Applied Social Sciences, The Hong Kong Polytechnic University, Room HJ407, Core H, Hunghom, Hong Kong. E-mail: danielshek@inet.polyu.edu.hk

attributes in inter-parental relationships. The developed measure is pioneering in both the Chinese and international contexts.

INTRODUCTION

Inter-parental relationship is an important determinant of adolescent development and mental health (1,2). A high level of inter-parental conflict and overt inter-parental violence are risk factors for both depression and aggression in adolescents (3,4). Moreover, inter-parental conflict was related to adolescent internalizing and externalizing disorders, conduct problems, poor peer interaction, poor health, depression, anxiety, attachment insecurity, and low self-esteem (1,5,6-12).

However, aside from conflict-related attributes, there are also non-conflict related attributes in the inter-parent relationship, such as the degree of care and concern, communication and mutuality. Unfortunately, compared with inter-parental conflict, very few studies have examined non-conflict related aspects of perceived marital quality from the perspective of adolescent children (i.e., inter-parental relationship perceived by adolescents). This area should be examined as there are studies showing that adolescents were influenced by the non-conflict related attributes of the relationship of their parents (13,14).

Conceptually, there are two problems of over-emphasis on inter-parental conflict. First, focusing on inter-parental conflict alone assumes a conflict orientation in the conception of inter-parental relationships. This orientation views the inter-parental relationship as a source of problem rather than a source of support within family system (i.e., pathological perspective). Second, focusing only on inter-parental conflict neglects the fact that inter-parental relationships are multi-dimensional. This might mask the possible contribution of different aspects of inter-parental relationships to adolescent development.

There are views suggesting that it is important to segregate positive and negative relationship characteristics of marriage and that such characteristics are separable (but related) dimensions of inter-parental relationships (15, 16). On one hand, negative aspects of interpersonal relationships, such as conflicts, complaints, criticism, hostility, withdrawal, and defensiveness differentiated distressed from non-distressed couples (17-19), have predicted divorce in newly married couples (20). These negative characteristics were associated with deterioration of marital satisfaction over time (21).On the other hand, positive aspects of interpersonal relationships, such as expressed warmth and support, have also been recognized as important indicators of relationship satisfaction (17,22,23), with lower rates of positive behavior characterizing distressed marriages (19).

There are theories suggesting that positive attributes of inter-parental relationships are related to adolescent developmental outcomes (24) and there is empirical support for some of such theoretical propositions. For example, greater positive affect in the inter-parental relationship was indirectly associated with fewer externalizing behavior problems in preschoolers via parenting behavior (25). However, little is known about whether positive inter-parental relationships can still predict unique adolescent mental health after controlling for negative inter-parental relationships.

Positive inter-parental relationships, including inter-parental non-conflict related attributes, might be particularly important for Chinese people because relationship harmony was emphasized in the Chinese culture (26). As conflict behavior is not easily expressed in

Chinese families (which may explain its low occurrence), inter-parental conflict may not be a sensitive indicator of inter-parental marital quality perceived by children (26). Therefore, to understand marital quality in terms of inter-parental relationship perceived by adolescent children, non-conflict related inter-parental relationship attributes should be examined.

It is necessary to understand adolescent perception of parental marital quality in terms of non-conflict related attributes for two obvious reasons. First, based on stress and coping theories (27-29), adolescents' own perception and interpretation of inter-parental relationships mediate the impacts of actual inter-parental relationship on adolescent developmental outcomes. In other words, adolescent perception of inter-parental relationships might affect how suchrelationships actually influence adolescent development (30). Second, adolescent perceptions and understanding of inter-parental relationships might be different from those of parents (30). Parental reports may be biased because children may be aware of negative inter-parental interaction to which they are not directly exposed to. For example, parents may not realize that their children overhear disagreements that take place in another room or after they have gone to bed. Parent reports may also under-estimate children's awareness of negative inter-parental interaction because parents may define some interactions, such as disagreements that are resolved quickly and calmly, as conflicts that are not salient to children. Therefore, measures that directly assess adolescent perceptions of conflict are likely to provide more accurate assessment of the quality of inter-parental relationship. Empirically, Joshi (31) showed that children's perceptions of inter-parental relationships aredifferent from those of parents, and the differences in perceptions aremoderated by gender of the children.

One of the most widely used and recognized measures of children's perceptions of inter-parental relationship is the Children's Perception of Inter-parental Conflict Scale (CPIC, 30). It was developed to assess children's view on their parents' conflict. Previous studies showed that the CPIC was applicable to adolescents and children in elementary schools . However, there has been no measure or assessment of positive aspects of inter-parental relationship from the perspectives ofthese two age groups. Moreover, there has been no validated Chinese scale assessing perceived marital quality of the parents from the perspective of adolescent children. To fill this research gap, a scale was constructed in this study to assess adolescent perception of the marital quality of their parents in terms of non-conflict related attributes in inter-parental relationships.

OUR STUDY

There were three steps in the construction of the new scale. The first step was item development which, was based on a thorough review of the literature on marital quality and assessment of inter-parental relationships and interactions. The second step was qualitative data collection via focus groups. Four focus group interviews with Chinese adolescents and social workers with family service experiences were carried out to generate items on marital quality perceived by adolescent children. The final step was to ascertain the content validity of the proposed items. Experts were invited to assess the content validity of the scale and to examine whether the items could be refined.

Step 1: Systematic literature review

The first step was to generate items based on previous literature on marital quality and measurement tools of marital relationship and interactions. Graham, Diebels and Barnow(32) pointed out several widely used marital quality measures, such as the Locke–Wallace Marital Adjustment Test, the Kansas Marital Satisfaction Scale, the Quality of Marriage Index, Relationship Assessment Scale, Marital Opinion Questionnaire, Karney and Bradbury's (21) semantic differential scale (SMD), and the Couples Satisfaction Index. The above scales were thoroughly reviewed. In addition, computer search via PsycINFO using various combinations of keywords (i.e., "relationship", "relationship satisfaction", "loves", "measure", "assessment", "measurement", and "tool") was carried out in August 2011. Articles not related to assessment tools on inter-parental relationship were removed. Finally, eight articles were identified (e.g., 33,34) and the Triangular Love Scale, Dyadic Adjustment Scale and Dyadic Trust Scale suggested by these articles were also reviewed. In the scales under review, items describing non-conflict related behaviors that might be observable to children were selected, and therepeated items were removed. The identified non-conflict related behaviors were then used to form items for adolescent children. Based on this step, an initial item pool of 32 items was tentatively developed.

Step 2: Focus group studies

Obviously, the items generated by literature review might not be extensively enough to cover adolescents' perception of inter-parental non-conflict related attributes, particularly within the Chinese culture. With the very limited literature in this area, it is essential to understand the phenomenon directly from the stakeholders. The process is of special importance for an indigenous study where cultural specificity is emphasized. Qualitative study allows researchers to grasp the native meanings and characteristics of the phenomenon, in order to make indigenous conceptualization of the phenomenon possible (35). Therefore, focus groups were used to explore adolescents' perception of the marital quality of their parents. In this study, two focus groups of adolescents and two focus groups of social workers with family services experiences were conducted and interviewed separately.

Participants and procedures

In this study, two focus groups of adolescents and two focus groups of social workers with family services experiences were conducted. The adolescents were recruited from a local secondary school whereas social workers with family services experiences were recruited from two family services units in Hong Kong. The first adolescent group consisted of 4 boys and 4 girls, with age ranged from 12 to 16 (M=12.93, SD=0.91). The second adolescent group consisted of 3 boys and 5 girls, with age ranged from 12 to 16 (M=12.13, SD=0.84). Three of them came from single parent families, while others came from intact families. Written consent from parents was obtained for the adolescents to join the focus group. The adolescents were requested to voice out their perception of their parents' relationship and interaction.

The first social worker group consisted of 5 social workers with at least 3 years working experiences in family services. The second social worker group consisted of 7 social workers with at least 2 years working experiences in family services. Two were male and 10 were female. Theirconsent was also obtained. Also, the social workers were requested to voice out their ideas and experiences on children's perception of inter-parental relationship attributes. The first author conducted both interviews and the processes were audio-recorded. Each focus group interviews of adolescents and social workers lasted about an hour. The interview guides of adolescents and social workers can be seen in Table 1 and 2.

Items were further developed based on the focus group interview findings. The findings of focus groups were summarized into themes. Examples from each theme were selected, and examples with similar meanings were re-written as items.

Step 3: Content validation by experts

While focus groups could yield rich information for the construction of the scale on adolescent perception of inter-parental non-conflicted related attributes, it is necessary to assess the content validity of the proposed measure. Content validity refers to the extent to which a measurement reflects the specific intended domain of the content (36). It is based on a detailed examination of the content of the test items. In this study, it includes reviewing the relevance of each item to the construct, the overall representativeness of test items, and the clarity of test item by experts (37).

Table 1. Interview guides of Adolescent focus groups

1	Is the relationship between your parents good?
2	Is the relationship between your parents good? Can you tell whether the relationship is good? How you can know?
3	When observing the relationship between your parents, what aspects will you pay attention to?
4	How would you define whether the relationship between your parents is good?
5	In addition to inter-parental conflicts, what else do you can use to judge whether the relationship between your parents is good?
6	Will you use "whether parents appreciate each other" as a way to judge their inter-parental relationship quality?
7	Is "inter-parental consistency in opinion, thinking and behaviors" a way to judge their inter-parental relationship quality?
8	Is "whether parents spend time together or share with each other" a way to judge their inter-parental relationship quality?
9	Is "inter-parental trust" a way to judge their inter-parental relationship quality?
10	Is "inter-parental respect" your way to judge their inter-parental relationship quality?

Participants and procedure

In this validation study, an expert panel (N = 21) was set up. Experts with at least one year of experience in providing social work or counseling services for families of adolescents or had substantial knowledge inter-parental relationship were invited to participate in the content validation process. Experts were invited if they could meet any of the following criteria:

(1) at least one year working experience in family services;
(2) substantial knowledge about the Chinese culture; and
(3) expertise in understanding the literacy level of secondary school students.

The panel consisted of 21 social workers who met all the proposed criteria. Regarding their experiences in family services, their mean working experiences was 12.33 years(SD=8.40). Regarding their educational levels, 5 experts had obtained a Master's degree, 15 experts had a Bachelor's degree and 1 expert got a diploma in the social work discipline.

As they reviewed the content validity of the developed items, the experts were required to examine:

(1) the relevance of the test items to the construct or subscales measured in the instruments;
(2) the representativeness of the items to a particular content domain (i.e., how far the domains cover all the facets of the targeted constructs), and
(3) the clarity of the test items(i.e., whether the wordings and phases were clear and concise).

A self-administered questionnaire was used to collect the opinion of the experts. The experts were informed of the definitions, related literature, domains of the construct, as well as the assessment items. They were requested to fill in the questionnaire reflecting their judgment of the content validity of the instruments. Regarding the "relevance" of the test items to the construct, a 4-point rating scale (1 = irrelevant, 2 = item is in need of revision or otherwise it would no longer be relevant, 3 = relevant but needs minor amendment, 4 = relevant) was used to measure how far each item was relevant to the content domain. Justifications were requested for items that were considered irrelevant, and recommendations on modifications of items that needed revision were also requested. Regarding the "clarity" of the items, a 4-point Likert scale (1 = very unclear, 2 = unclear, 3 = clear, 4 = very clear) was used to see whether the wordings and phases were concise and clearly presented. Again, recommendations on modifications of the wordings and phases were requested in case an item was perceived as unclearly presented. For the "representativeness" of items to the domains, a 4-point Likert scale (1 = very inadequate, 2= inadequate, 3 = adequate, 4 = very adequate) was used to evaluate how far the items cover the facets of the domains. Recommendations were asked if the items were considered under-represented. Overall, the representativeness of the domains with reference to the targeted construct and the representativeness of the scale as a whole were also evaluated by a 4-point Likert scale. An open-ended question was used to examine the overall representativeness of the domains in covering the different facets of the targeted construct.

FINDINGS

The content of the focus groups was fully transcribed and pattern coding was carried out. Miles and Huberman(38) suggested that pattern coding is a way of grouping similar content of focus groups into a small number of sets, themes, or constructs. Four focus groups were coded by two coders. One was a PhD student of applied social sciences. The second was a registered social worker with a Master's degree in social work. The coding scheme was developed by the first coder after he had read all the transcripts twice. The second coder coded the transcripts by using the coding scheme developed by the first coder. The inter-rater reliabilities for social worker focus groups were .93 and .91, whereas those for adolescent focus groups were. 89, and .88 respectively. The inter-rater reliabilities for social worker focus group were a bit higher than those for adolescent our focus groups

Analyses of the content of the four focus groups showed that fourteen themes (i.e., respect, appreciation, responsibility, trust, body touch, togetherness, intimacy, communication, acceptance, concern, criticism, consistency, helping, and response) emerged from the data. Table 3 lists the themes of adolescent perception of non-conflict related attributes in inter-parental relationships.

The findings of the focus groups provided some insights into adolescents' perception of inter-parental non-conflict related attributes. Apart from the dimensions of trust, intimacy, communication, criticism, and respect, other domains such as togetherness, responsibility, appreciation, response, body touch, consistency and helping had been experienced and were mentioned by the adolescents.

Table 2. Interview guides of Social worker focus groups

1	Based on your working experiences, what are the characteristics of a good marital relationship?
2	How can you tell whether a couple is having a good relationship?
3	What is the behavior expression of a couple having a good relationship?
4	How can you know whether a couple will not divorce?
5	Can children know whether their parents are having a good relationship? If they can know, how can they know?
6	What aspect will children observe when judging their parents' relationship?
7	What do you think about adolescents' perception on their parents' relationship?
8	How does Chinese culture define a good marital relationship?
9	In Chinese culture, what is a good marital relationship?
10	Present literature of inter-parental relationship focus on conflicts, In addition to conflicts, what else can be used to judge whether the relationship between parents is good?

Both adolescents and social workers mentioned "togetherness" and "communication" as important and observable indicators of inter-parental relationship quality. Both groups shared in detail how they perceived togetherness and communication serve as signs of having a positive inter-parental relationship. While social workers emphasized the importance of acceptance, adolescents did not emphasize the importance of this attribute. In addition, the participating adolescents did not regard acceptance as a behavioral expression of a positive inter-parental relationship. Adolescents reported that they felt uneasy expressing their perception of their parents' relationships and interactions. As a result, they spoke less when compared with social worker focus groups.

Based on the focus group findings, indigenous items measuring adolescent perception of inter-parental non-conflict related attributes was generated. An item pool was developed by both literature review and the results of focus groups. From the item pool, repeated items were removed and 60 items finally remained. Based on item content similarity, they were re-organized into 12 domains, namely Togetherness, Communication, Appreciation, Criticism, Concern, Helping, Understanding and Acceptance, Trust, Satisfaction, Indigenous Chinese concepts, Passion, and Commitment. The 60 items are presented in Table 4.

Content validation study

The evaluation of content validity of the measure was performed using two analytical strategies:

(1) calculation of Content Validity Index (CVI) on aspect of relevance, clarity and representativeness, and
(2) analysis of feedback and recommendations of the experts for the improvement of the items and the scale.

Regarding the calculation of CVI, the method suggested by Rubio et al. (39) was used. The method was to compute the CVI of each item by counting the number of experts who rated positively (3 or 4) on the evaluation aspect of the item and then dividing the number by the total number of experts. This provided a measure of the proportion of experts who considered the item as valid. The CVI for the measure was estimated by calculating the average CVI across the items. A CVI of .80 was recommended as the indicator for content validity for new measures (40).

Aside from CVI, experts were asked to give feedback on the justifications of the "poorly designed" items, as well as recommendations for improvement of the items and the scales. Analysis of content was made to understand the feedback of the scales. The overall CVIs on relevance, clarity and representativeness were .92, .89 and .90 respectively, showing that the scale has good content validity in the aspects of relevance, clarity and representativeness.

Table 3. Themes of adolescents' perception of inter-parental non-conflict related attributes

Themes	Examples of Narratives	No. of participants mentioned		
		Adolescent	Social worker	Total
Respect	"(Father) will listen to mother's opinion when deciding things" (S, a 12-year-old girl)	7	19	26
Appreciation	"My father will praise my mom if she cooks good food" (M, a 13-year-old girl)	7	38	45
Responsibility	"My mother said…my father is very responsible…taking care of the family…" (M, a 13-year-old girl)	11	49	60
Trust	"Trust…can make the relationship survive in time…the kids might know…" (G, a female social workers)	5	2	7
Body touch	"They (parents) holding hands…"(L, a 13-year-old girl) "They (parents) kiss in front of me…" (W, a 13-year-old boy)	8	8	16
Togetherness	"I feel their relationship is good and secured if they (parents sit down on the sofa and watch TV together" (J, a 13-year-old girl) "They (parents) cook together…feel that they are close…"(H, 11-year-old boy)	49	41	90
Intimacy	"My father will miss my mom. He will call her once he is off from work" (L, a 13-year-old girl)	8	9	17
Communication	"I observe whether they (the parents) talk to each other before sleeping to judge if their relationship is good" (K, a 12-year-old boy)	48	31	79
Acceptance	"Accept each other's weakness…even the mother is in bad mood…the father accept it and focus her sacrifice for the family…"(A, a female social worker)	0	12	12
Concern	"(Mother) tell him (the father) to get more cloths when it is cold" (M, a 13-year-old girl)	15	28	43
Criticism	"(Father) say bad things about her (mother)" (L, a 13-year-old girl)	20	25	45
Consistency	"They will act the same ways and do not allow me to…when their relationship is good" (K, a 12-year-old boy)	4	20	24
Helping	"Helping…is a sign of good relationship and bonding" (B, a 12-year-old boy)	12	11	23
Response	"My mom knows what is in my dad's mind…understand his behaviors…she will give him slippers automatically without my dad saying anything" (H, 11-year-old boy)	1	15	16
Total		195	308	503

Table 4. 60-item pool of adolescents' perception of inter-parental non-conflict related attributes

	A: Togetherness(Yi-Qi)
1.	My parents do things together.
2.	My parents stay at home together.
3.	In their spare time, my parents took me out together.
4.	When my parents are at home, they do their own things.
5.	When my parents are at home, they rarely work together.
	B: Communication (Gou-Tong)
6.	My parents talk to each other and share fun.
7.	My parents share little things in life with each other.
8.	My parents talk to each other when having dinner.
9.	My parents get along well.
10.	My parents have communication.
11	My parents are in a Cold War.
12.	My parents ignore each other.
13.	My parents communicate with a good attitude.
14.	My parents know each other well.
	C: Appreciation (Xin-Shang)
15.	My parents affirm each other's contribution to the family.
16.	My parents praise each other.
17.	My parents express that the other party is a good partner.
18.	My parents express that the other party is a good parent.
19.	My parents express their appreciation of each other
20.	My parents express that the other party is a responsible partner.
21.	My parents express that the other party is a responsible parent.
	D: Criticism(Pi-Ping)
22.	My parents say "bad things" about each other.
23.	My parents criticize each other.
24.	My parents express their complaints about each other.
25.	My parents expressed dissatisfaction with each other in front of me.
	E: Concern (Guan-Xin-Guan-Zhu)
26.	My parents care about each other.
27.	My parents are considerate of each other.
28.	My parents value each other.
29.	My parents respect each other.
30.	My parents take into account each other's views when making the decision.
	F: Helping(Bang-Zhu)
31.	My parents help each other.
32.	My parents show dissatisfaction when helping each other.
33.	My parents actively help when the other parties face difficulties.
34.	My parents expect their spouses to help when facing difficulties.
	G: (Understanding and Acceptance(Li-Jie-Bao-Rong)
35.	My parents accept their spouse's shortcomings.
36.	My parents tolerate their spouse's shortcomings.
37.	My parents understand their spouses' behavior.
38.	My parents have a tacit understanding of each other

	H:Trust(Shen-Ren)
39.	My parents say that their spouses cannot be trusted.
40.	My parents say that their spouses are completely honest.
41.	My parents express trust in each other.
42.	My parents say that the other's promise is credible.
	I: Satisfaction(Man-Yi)
43.	My parents are happy to get along.
44.	My parents' relationship is good.
45.	My parents are satisfied with their marriage.
46.	My parents are satisfied with each other.
47.	My parents have a good link between them,
48.	My parents will choose each other again if they had an opportunity to do so.
49.	My parents feel that the other is the ideal companion.
50.	My parents have confidence in each other.
51.	I hear that my parents express their regret in getting married.
	J: Indigenous Chinese concepts(Hua-Ren-She-Hui-GaiNian)
52.	My parents are courteous to each other as they are to guests.
53.	My parents "ren-i".
	K: Passion(Ji-Qing)
54.	My parents feel the other party is attractive.
55.	My parents' relationship is romantic.
56.	My parents adore each other.
	L: Commitment(Cheng-Nuo)
57.	My parents strain at their relationship.
58.	My parents committed to maintaining their relationship.
59.	My parents are confident in the stability of their relationship.
60.	My parents have a sense of responsibility for their marriage.

All items had $CVI_{(relevance)}$ greater than .80. Among the 60 items, 14 items obtained the $CVI_{(relevance)}$ of 1.0, indicating that all experts agreed the items appropriately described the measured construct. For clarity of the items and the scale, all items had $CVI_{(clarity)}$ greater than .80, suggesting a good validity value of the items in terms of clarity. The $CVI_{(clarity)}$ ranged from .81 to 1.0. There were 7 out of 60 items with $CVI_{(clarity)}$ value equaled to 1.0, indicating that all experts agreed that the items were clearly presented. For representativeness, although 7 experts failed to report this part of information, the ratings from the remaining 14 experts showed that all 12 domains (Togetherness, Communication, Appreciation, Criticism, Concern, Helping, Understanding and Acceptance, Trust, Satisfaction, Indigenous Chinese concepts, Passion, and Commitment.) had $CVI_{(representativeness)}$ greater than .86, showing good content validity of the items in representing the domains. Furthermore, the calculated overall $CVI_{(representativeness)}$from 13 experts (i.e., 8 experts failed to provide this part of information) was 1.0. Also, the $CVI_{(representativeness)}$ of the scale rated by experts was .90. Both ratings suggested that the scale obtained a good degree of representativeness of the measured construct. Tables 5 and 6 illustrate the overall CVI of the measure on aspects of relevance, clarity and representativeness.

Experts also gave feedback and suggestions on how the items could be improved. The experts regarded three items were not clear enough for early adolescents. Modifications of items are illustrated in Table 7.

Table 5. CVIon the measure on aspects of relevance, clarity and representativeness

Domain/Item			
A: Togetherness(Yi-Qi)	$CVI_{(relevance)}$	$CVI_{(clarity)}$	$CVI_{(representativeness)}$
01	.95	.90	1.00
02	.95	.81	.90
03	.86	.86	.90
04	.90	.86	.81
05	1.00	.86	.90
A: Togetherness(Yi-Qi) Average	.93	.86	.90
B: Communication (Gou-Tong)	$CVI_{(relevance)}$	$CVI_{(clarity)}$	$CVI_{(representativeness)}$
06	1.00	1.00	1.00
07	1.00	1.00	1.00
08	.95	.95	.95
09	1.00	.95	1.00
10	1.00	.95	.95
11	.90	.81	.90
12	.90	.90	.90
13	1.00	1.00	1.00
14	1.00	.95	.95
B: Communication (Gou-Tong) Average	.97	.95	.96
C: Appreciation (Xin-Shang)	$CVI_{(relevance)}$	$CVI_{(clarity)}$	$CVI_{(representativeness)}$
15	.90	.90	.90
16	.86	.86	.86
17	.90	.90	.90
18	.90	.86	.90
19	.86	.81	.86
20	.90	.86	.90
21	.90	.90	.90
C: Appreciation (Xin-Shang) Average	.89	.87	.89
D: Criticism (Pi-Ping)	$CVI_{(relevance)}$	$CVI_{(clarity)}$	$CVI_{(representativeness)}$
22	.86	.81	.86
23	.95	.90	.95
24	.90	.81	.90
25	.90	.86	.90
D: Criticism (Pi-Ping) Average	.90	.85	.90
E: Concern (Guan-Xin-Guan-Zhu)	$CVI_{(relevance)}$	$CVI_{(clarity)}$	$CVI_{(representativeness)}$
26	1.00	.90	.90
27	.95	.86	.86
28	1.00	.90	.90
29	.95	.86	.86
30	1.00	.90	.90

Domain/Item			
E: Concern(Guan-Xin-Guan-Zhu) Average	.98	.88	.88
F: Helping (Bang-Zhu)	$CVI_{(relevance)}$	$CVI_{(clarity)}$	$CVI_{(representativeness)}$
31	1.00	1.00	1.00
32	.90	.90	.90
33	.90	.90	.90
34	.90	.90	.86
F: Helping (Bang-Zhu) Average	.93	.93	.92
G: (Understanding and Acceptance (Li-Jie-Bao-Rong)	$CVI_{(relevance)}$	$CVI_{(clarity)}$	$CVI_{(representativeness)}$
35	.90	.81	.86
36	.90	.86	.90
37	.90	.81	.90
38	1.00	1.00	.95
G: (Understanding and Acceptance (Li-Jie-Bao-Rong) Average	.93	.87	.90
H:Trust(Shen-Ren)	$CVI_{(relevance)}$	$CVI_{(clarity)}$	$CVI_{(representativeness)}$
39	.90	.86	.90
40	.90	.81	.86
41	.90	.86	.90
42	.90	.86	.90
H:Trust(Shen-Ren) Average	.90	.85	.89
I: Satisfaction (Man-Yi)	$CVI_{(relevance)}$	$CVI_{(clarity)}$	$CVI_{(representativeness)}$
43	1.00	1.00	1.00
44	1.00	1.00	1.00
45	.90	.86	.90
46	.90	.86	.86
47	.90	.90	.86
48	.90	.86	.86
49	.90	.90	.90
50	.81	.81	.81
51	.90	.86	.86
I: Satisfaction (Man-Yi) Average	.91	.89	.89
J: Indigenous Chinese concepts (Hua-Ren-She-Hui-GaiNian)	$CVI_{(relevance)}$	$CVI_{(clarity)}$	$CVI_{(representativeness)}$
52	.86	.90	.86
53	.86	.95	.81
J: Indigenous Chinese concepts (Hua-Ren-She-Hui-GaiNian) Average	.86	.93	.84
K:Passion (Ji-Qing)	$CVI_{(relevance)}$	$CVI_{(clarity)}$	$CVI_{(representativeness)}$
54	.86	.90	.90
55	.95	.95	.81

Table 5. (Continued)

Domain/Item			
56	.95	.95	.95
K:Passion (Ji-Qing) Average	.92	.93	.89
L:Commitment (Cheng-Nuo)	$CVI_{(relevance)}$	$CVI_{(clarity)}$	$CVI_{(representativeness)}$
57	.90	.81	.86
58	.90	.86	.90
59	.90	.90	.90
60	.90	.86	.86
L:Commitment (Cheng-Nuo) Average	.90	.86	.88
Overall Average	.92	.89	.90

DISCUSSION

With reference to the limited literature on the theoretical conceptualization of adolescent perception of inter-parental non-conflict related attributes, the paper presents findings on the conceptualization of this construct in the Chinese culture as well as evidence of content validity of the measure, which is considered as pioneering in this area both in the Chinese and international contexts.

The findings based on the focus groups with adolescents and social workers suggested that adolescents' perception on inter-parental relationships went beyond trust, intimacy, communication, criticism, and respect as suggested by the conventional literature on marital satisfaction and stability. The findings suggest that physical togetherness of parents, responsibility shared by parents for the family, appreciation expressed in front of children, active response to partners' needs, body touch, consistency in term of views and behaviors of parents, and active helping are important constructs to be considered. These domains enrich the theoretical conceptualization of adolescents' perception on inter-parental relationship, especially in the Hong Kong Chinese context.

The present study also showed discrepancies in the perceptions of adolescents and social workers. It pointed out the differences between "non-expert" and "expert" in understanding long-term committed relationship. For instance, in the domain of acceptance and responsibility, social workers emphasized acceptance. In contrast, adolescents did not report that acceptance of each other's weakness was an important attribute. Neither did adolescents regard acceptance as a behavioral expression of positive inter-parental relationships. For the theme "responsibility", although adolescents also reported they had observed their parents being responsible for their families and regarded responsibility as a behavioral expression of positive inter-parental relationship, their tendency of reporting this domain was relatively lower than that of social workers. These two differences might be due to the fact that adolescents had less experience in a long-term romantic relationship and they were still unable to appreciate the importance of acceptance and responsibility in such a relationship. Alternatively, this can be explained by the influence of popular youth culture (i.e., its emphases on lust and feelings in intimate relationships) on contemporary young people.

The content validation done by experts showed that the measure had good content validity in the aspects of relevance, clarity and representativeness. This step was important as it ensured that the items developed were valid from the perspectives of the judges. The modification of the items based on the views of the judges further improved the validity of the measure. The present study has three implications. First, the study contributes to the conceptualization of inter-parental non-conflict related attributes from the perspective of adolescents. The domains and themes of adolescent perception of inter-parental non-conflict related attributes derived from the focus groups underscore the importance of investigating various aspects of inter-parental relationships, such as physical togetherness and appreciation. Second, this study helps to formulate and develop an indigenous measurement tool that can facilitate our further exploration of indigenous Chinese concepts as well as construction of family models applicable to Chinese people. Third, development of the measurement tool may bring special value for further research on the association between inter-parental relationship and adolescents' development. Previous studies on the association between inter-parental relationships and adolescents' development focused on parental conflict (1, 2), with little attention paid to positive aspects of inter-parental relationships, such as non-conflict related attributes. The proposed measure developed in this study makes it possible to examine the unique contribution of different aspects of inter-parental relationship to adolescent development. It also helps social workers enhance adolescent mental health by teaching those skills that foster inter-parental non-conflict related attributes, such as active response to partners' need and appreciation.

Table 6. $CVI_{(representativeness)}$ of 12 domains with reference to adolescent perception on inter-parental non-conflict related attributes*

Domain	$CVI_{(representativeness)}$
A: Togetherness(Yi-Qi)	.93
B: Communication (Gou-Tong)	.93
C: Appreciation(Xin-Shang)	.93
D: Criticism (Pi-Ping)	.93
E: Concern (Guan-Xin-Guan-Zhu)	.86
F: Helping (Bang-Zhu)	.93
G: Understanding and Acceptance (Li-Jie-Bao-Rong)	.86
H: Trust (Shen-Ren)	.86
I: Satisfaction (Man-Yi)	.86
J: Indigenous Chinese concepts (Hua-Ren-She-Hui-GaiNian)	.86
K: Passion (Ji-Qing)	.86
L: Commitment (Cheng-Nuo)	.93
Overall Average	.90

* The ratings were given by 14 experts as 7 experts did not respond the items.

The present study has several limitations. First, qualitative findings based on the focus groups may have the inherit limitation of generalizability. Second, the adolescent sample was mainly confined to early adolescents, resulting in over-representation of younger adolescents' perception of the construct and under-representation of the views of older adolescents. Third, the use of focus group may hinder the participant's involvement, as the adolescents tended to restrain themselves when reporting in a group. Perhaps they felt unnatural to talk about their perception of inter-parental relationship and interaction publicly. Adolescents' hesitation in reporting might explain why they spoke less than social workers. Their anxiety in mentioning their parents' behavior might also explain why the data of the adolescent focus groups were a little less consistent than those of social worker focus groups as indexed by inter-rater reliability statistics. Fourth, as the findings presented in the study were based on adolescents and social workers in Hong Kong, there is a need to assess the generalizability of the findings in different Chinese communities (e.g. mainland China and Taiwan).

Despite the above limitations, this study can be considered as pioneering in exploring adolescent perception of inter-parental non-conflict related attributes and in development of a measure that is indigenous in the Chinese context. The measure was based on qualitative data of social workers and adolescents and validated by a panel of experts. Essentially, the study can be regarded as positive response to the urge on "open(ing) new paths to a deeper understanding of Chinese cultural, social, and psychological processes and patterns" (p. 182, 35). In addition, as there are few validated psychosocial measures in different Chinese societies (41-44), the present study is an important addition to the literature.

Table 7. Modifications of the scale of adolescents' perception of inter-parental non-conflict related attributes

Item	Problem and suggestions made	Modifications
19. My parents appreciate each other	Two experts thought that appreciation might not be a publicly observable behavioral expression	The item was changed to "My parents express their appreciation of each other".
24. My parents complain each other	Two experts thought that complaint might not be a publicly observable behavioral expression	The item was changed to "My parents express their complaint of each other".
33. My parents will help when the other parties face difficulties	Three experts thought that inter-parental helping might be unwilling under some situations and unwilling helping cannot reflect positive inter-parental relationship	The item was changed to "My parents actively help when the other parties face difficulties".

REFERENCES

[1] Cumming, EM, Davies, PT. The impact of parents on their children: An emotional security perspective. Ann Child Dev 1995;10:167-208.

[2] Cummings, EM, Davies, PT. Effects of marital conflict on children: Recent advances and emerging themes in process-oriented research. J Child Psychol Psychiatry 2002; 43:31-63.

[3] Conger, RD, Conger, KJ, Elder, GH, Lorenz, FO. (1992). A family process model of economic hardship and adjustment of early adolescent boys. Child Dev 1992; 63: 526–41.

[4] Cowan, PA, Cowan, CP. Interventions as tests of family systems theories: Marital and family relationships in children's development and psychopathology. Dev Psycho pathol 2002; 14: 731–59.

[5] Rutter, M. Sex differences in response to family stress. In Anthony EJ. Koupernik,C. The child in his family. New York: Wiley, 1970: 165-96.

[6] Grych, JH, Fincham, FD. (1990). Marital conflict and children's adjustment: A cognitive-contextual framework. Psychol Bull 1990; 108:267-90.
[7] Emery, RE. Marriage, divorce, and children's adjustment, 2nd ed. Thousand Oaks, CA: Sage, 1999.
[8] Gottman, JM, Katz, LF. Effects of marital discord on young children's peer interactions and health. DevPsychol 1989;25:273-81.
[9] Howes, P. Markman, HJ. Marital quality and child attachment: A longitudinal study, Child Dev 1989;60:1044-51.
[10] Jouriles, EN, Bourg, WJ, Farris, AM. Marital adjustment and child conduct problems: A comparison of the correlation across subsamples. J Consult Clin Psychol 1991;59:354-7.
[11] Katz, LF, Gottman, JM. Patterns of marital conflict predict children's internalizing and externalizing behaviors. Dev Psychol 1993; 29(6): 940-50.
[12] Amato, PA, Sobolewski, JM. The Effects of Divorce and Marital Discord on Adult Children's Well-Being. Am Sociol Rev 2001;66(6):900-21.
[13] Feldman, SS, Fisher, L, Seitel, L. A longitudinal study of the effects of parents' marital satisfaction on the adaptation of young adults. JRes Adolesc 1997;7: 55-80.
[14] Hair, EC, Moore, KA, Hadley, AM, Keyes, K, Day, RD, Orthner, DK. Parent marital quality and the parent–adolescent relationship: Effects on adolescent and young adult health outcomes. Marriage FamRev 2009;45(2-3):218-48.
[15] Kiecolt-Glaser, JK, Newton, TL. Marriage and health: His and hers. Psychol Bull 2001;127(4):472-503.
[16] Whisman, MA. The association between depression and marital dissatisfaction. InBeach S. R. H. Marital and family processes in depression: A scientific foundation for clinical practice Washington, DC: American Psychological Association, 2001:3-24.
[17] Fincham, FD. Marital conflict: Correlates, structure and context. Curr Dir Psychol Sci 2003;12:23-7.
[18] Matthews, L, Wickrama, KAS, Conger, RD. Predicting marital instability from spouse and observer reports of marital interaction. J Marriage Fam 1996;58:641-55.
[19] Snyder, D, Heyman, R, Haynes, S. Evidence-based approaches to assessing couple distress. Psychol Assess 2005;17:288-307.
[20] Gottman, J. What predicts divorce? The relationship between marital processes and marital outcomes. Hillsdale, NJ: Lawrence Erlbaum, 1994.
[21] Karney, BR, Bradbury, TN. Neuroticism, marital interaction, and the trajectory of marital satisfaction. J Pers Soc Psychol 1997;72:1075–92.
[22] Pasch, LA, Bradbury, TN. Social support, conflict, and the development of marital dysfunction. J Consult Clin Psychol 1998;66:219–30.
[23] Sarason, IG, Pierce, GR, Sarason, BR. General and specific perceptions of social support. In Avison WR, Gotlib IH. Stress and mental health: Contemporary issues and prospects for thefuture. New York: Plenum Press, 1994:151-77.
[24] Frosch, CA, **Mangelsdorf**, SC, McHale, JL. Marital behavior and the security of preschooler-parent attachment relationships. J Fam Psychol 2000;14:144-61.
[25] Miller, NB, Cowan, PA, Cowan, CP, Hetherington, EM, Clingempeel, WG. Externalizing in preschoolers and early adolescents: A cross-study replication of a family model. Dev Psychol 1993;29:3-18.
[26] Shek, DTL. Parental Marital Quality and Well-Being, Parent-Child Relational Quality, and Chinese Adolescent Adjustment. Am J FamTher 2000;28:147–62.
[27] Compas, BE. Stress and life events during childhood and adolescence. Clin Psychol Rev 1987;7:275-302.
[28] Lazarus, RS, Folkman, S. Stress, Appraisal, and Coping. New York: Springer, 1984.
[29] Rutter, M. (1983). Stress, coping and development: some issues and some questions. In Garmezy, N, RutterM. Ctr for Advanced Study in the Behavioral Sciences. New York: McGraw-Hill, 1983:1-41.
[30] Grych, JH, Seid, M, Fincham, FD. Assessing marital conflict from the child's perspective: The Children's Perception of Interparental Conflict Scale. *Child Dev 1992;* 63:558–72.
[31] Joshi, A. Parents' and children's perceptions of interparental conflict resolution. PsycholRep 2001;88(3):943-6.

[32] Graham, JM, Diebels, KJ, Barnow, ZB. The reliability of relationship satisfaction: a reliability generalization Meta-analysis. J FamPsychol 2011; 25(1):39-48.
[33] Graham, JM, Christiansen, K. The reliability of romantic love: A reliability generalizationmeta-analysis. Pers Relatsh 2009;16:49-66.
[34] Graham, JM, Liu, YJ, Jeziorski, JL. The Dyadic Adjustment Scale: A reliabilitygeneralizability meta-analysis. J Marriage Fam 2006;68: 701-17.
[35] Yang KS. Towards an indigenous Chinese psychology: A selective review of methodological, theoretical, and empirical accomplishments. Chinese J Psychol 1999;41(2):181-211.
[36] Reber, A.S. Penguin dictionary of psychology. London: Penguin books, 1995.
[37] Rubin, A, Babbie, E. Essential research methods for social work. Belmont, CA: Thomson Brooks Cole, 2007.
[38] Miles, MB, Huberman, AM. Qualitative data analysis. Thousand Oaks. CA: Sage, 1994.
[39] Rubio, DM, Berg-Weger, M, Tebb, SS, Lee, ES, Rauch, S. Objectifying content validity: Conducting a content validity in social work research. Soc Work Res 2003; 27(2):94-104.
[40] Davi, L. Instrument review: Getting the most from your panel of experts. Appl Nurs Res 1992; 5:194-7.
[41] Leung JTY, Shek DTL. Validation of the Chinese Parental Expectation on Child's Future Scale. Int J Disabil. Human Dev 2011;10(3): 267-74.
[42] Shek DTL. Quality of life research: Responses to emerging issues in a changing world. Soc Indic Res 2011;100:371-74.
[43] Shek DTL, Yu L. A review of validated youth prevention and positive youth development programs in Asia. Int J Adolesc Med Health 2011; 23:317-24.
[44] Shek DTL, Ma HK, Sun RCF. A brief overview of adolescent developmental problems in Hong Kong. Scientific World Journal 2011;11:2243-56.

INTRAPERSONAL DEVELOPMENT AND LEADERSHIP

In: Chinese Adolescent Development ISBN: 978-1-62618-622-4
Editors: Daniel TL Shek, Rachel CF Sun, Joav Merrick © 2013 Nova Science Publishers, Inc.

Chapter 7

SECOND PILOTING OF A LEADERSHIP AND INTRAPERSONAL DEVELOPMENT SUBJECT AT THE HONG KONG POLYTECHNIC UNIVERSITY

Daniel TL Shek*[1], Rachel CF Sun[2], Walter WH Yuen[1], Yat H Chui[1], Allen Dorcas[1], Cecilia MS Ma[1], Lu Yu[1], Yammy LY Chak[1], Moon YM Law[1], Yida YH Chung[1] and Pik Fong Tsui[1]

[1]The Hong Kong Polytechnic University, Hong Kong, PRC
[2]The University of Hong Kong, Hong Kong, PRC

ABSTRACT

At The Hong Kong Polytechnic University, a course entitled "Tomorrow's Leaders" focusing on positive youth development constructs was developed for the students admitted under the New Undergraduate Curriculum in 2012/13 academic year to fulfill the requirement of "Leadership and Intrapersonal Development" under the General University Requirements. The subject was piloted in 2010/11 school year with very positive evaluation results. To refine the subject and to accumulate more experience, the subject was offered again in the first term of 2011/12 school year. The course content, evaluation strategies, and some initial findings based on the second piloting exercise are presented in this chapter. Consistent with the first piloting exercise, evaluation findings based on different strategies generally showed that the subject was able to promote the holistic development of students taking this subject.

INTRODUCTION

In response to the developmental needs of university students, all students under the New Undergraduate Curriculum at The Hong Kong Polytechnic University will be required to take

* Correspondence: Professor Daniel T.L. Shek, PhD, FHKPS, BBS, JP, Chair Professor of Applied Social Sciences, Faculty of Health and Social Sciences, Department of Applied Social Sciences, The Hong Kong Polytechnic University, Room HJ407, Core H, Hunghom, Hong Kong. E-mail: daniel.shek@polyu.edu.hk

a subject in the area of "Leadership and Intrapersonal Development" under the General University Requirements. With reference to this requirement, a subject entitled "Tomorrow's Leaders" was developed. Based on the literature on positive youth development and leadership, the subject attempts to nurture the development of students in the areas of self-understanding and interpersonal relationships with specific reference to leadership. The proposed course was piloted in the second term of 2010/11 academic year, with very favourable evaluation results. To further refine the subject and to accumulate more teaching experiences, the subject was piloted again in the first term of 2011/12 academic year. This chapter outlines the unique features of this course as well as the evaluation strategies adopted. Some initial evaluation findings of the second piloting exercise are also presented in this chapter.

"Tomorrow's leaders" at the Hong Kong Polytechnic University

To enable students to fulfill the "Leadership and Intrapersonal Development" requirement under the General University Requirements, the subject attempts to help students to understand themselves and maintain positive interpersonal relationships with reference to the qualities of effective leaders. It is expected that students can develop a higher level of awareness and understand the qualities of effective leaders after taking this subject. The objectives of the course and the intended learning outcomes can be seen in Table 1. To help students develop their personal qualities, subject matter on positive youth development constructs such as psychosocial competencies, resilience, interpersonal communication, and conflict resolution are included. The syllabus of the subject and the class schedule can be seen in Table 2 and Table 3, respectively.

Table 1. Objectives and learning outcomes of the subject

Objectives
1. To enable students to learn and integrate theories, research and concepts of the basic personal qualities (particularly intrapersonal and interpersonal qualities) of effective leaders; 2. To train students to develop and reflect on their intrapersonal and interpersonal qualities; 3. To promote the development of an active pursuit of knowledge on personal qualities in leadership amongst students.
Learning Outcomes
On successfully completing this subject, students will be able to: 1. understand and integrate theories, research and concepts on the basic qualities (particularly intrapersonal and interpersonal qualities) of effective leaders in the Chinese context; 2. develop self-awareness and understanding of oneself; 3. acquire interpersonal skills; 4. develop self-reflection skills in their learning; and 5. recognize the importance of an active pursuit of knowledge on intrapersonal and interpersonal leadership qualities.

Because the subject focuses on intrapersonal and interpersonal development, students taking this subject are expected to develop high sensitivity about their own behavior in the intrapersonal and interpersonal contexts. Besides, because this is a credit-bearing subject, intellectual thinking is emphasized in the subject, together with focus on experiential learning. Besides lectures which were designed to enable students to understand theories, concepts, and research on leadership qualities, simulation exercises, games, discussions, and case studies were carried out in the classroom context. Regarding the teaching and learning methodology, lectures, experiential learning sessions, group project presentations, and written assignments were used.

Table 2. Syllabus of the subject

Topic	Subject Content
1	An overview of the personal attributes of effective leaders: role of self-understanding and interpersonal relationship qualities. Required reading: Hogan, R., & Kaiser, R. B. (2005). What we know about leadership. *Review of General Psychology, 9*(2), 169-180.
2	Self-understanding: personality traits conducive to successful leadership. Required reading: Shek, D. T. L. (2010). Nurturing holistic development of university students in Hong Kong: Where are we and where should we go? *The Scientific World JOURNAL, 10*, 563-575.
3	Emotional competence: awareness and understanding of emotions, emotional quotient (EQ), role of emotional management in effective leadership, and mental health. Required reading: Lau, P. S. Y. (2006). Emotional competence as a positive youth development construct: Conceptual bases and implications for curriculum development. *International Journal of Adolescent Medicine and Health, 18*(3), 355-362.
4	Cognitive competence: different types of thinking, higher-order thinking, experiential learning, role of cognitive competence in effective leadership, and effective leaders as teachers. Required reading: Moseley, D., Elliott, J., Gregson, M., & Higgins, S. (2005). Thinking skills frameworks for use in education and training. *British Educational Research Journal, 31*(3), 367-390.
5	Resilience: stresses faced by adolescents, life adversities, coping with life stresses, adversity quotient (AQ), and role of resilience in effective leadership. Required reading: Lee, T. Y. (2006). Resilience as a positive youth development construct: Conceptual bases and implications for curriculum development. *International Journal of Adolescent Medicine and Health, 18*(3), 475-482.
6	Spirituality: meaning in life and adolescent development, spirituality and mental health, role of spirituality in effective leadership, and servant leadership. Required reading: Lau, P. S. Y. (2006). Spirituality as a positive youth development construct: Conceptual bases and implications for curriculum development. *International Journal of Adolescent Medicine and Health, 18*(3), 363-370.
7	Ethics and morality: moral issues and moral competence, role of ethics and morality in effective leadership, integrity and responsibility and effective leadership. Required readings: (i) Park, N., & Peterson, C. (2009). Character strengths: Research and practice. *Journal of College and Character, 10*(4), 1-10(ii) Dalton, J., & Crosby, P. (2007). Being and having: Shouldn't excellence in higher education (and people) be a measure of what one does rather than what one has? *Journal of College and Character, 9*(1), 1-5.

Table 2. (Continued)

Topic	Subject Content
8	Social competence: basic social competence skills, ability to build up positive human relationship, role of social competence in effective leadership, and egocentric mentality as a block to effective leadership. Required reading: Ma, H. K. (2006). Social competence as a positive youth development construct: Conceptual bases and implications for curriculum development. *International Journal of Adolescent Medicine and Health, 18*(3), 379-385.
9	Positive and healthy identity: self-identity, self-esteem and self-concept, self-discrepancies, role of self-concept in leadership, and self-leadership. Required reading: Tsang, S. K. M., & Yip, F. Y. Y. (2006). Positive identity as a positive youth development construct: Conceptual bases and implications for curriculum development. *International Journal of Adolescent Medicine and Health, 18*(3), 459-466.
10	Interpersonal communication: theories, concepts and skills of interpersonal communication, and role of communication skills in effective leadership. Required reading: de Vries, R. E., Bakker-Pieper, A., Siberg, R. A., van Gameren, K., & Vlug, M. (2009). The content and dimensionality of communication styles. *Communication Research, 36*, 178-206.
11	Interpersonal conflict; role of conflict resolution in effective leadership; team building; relationship quality and effective leadership. Required reading: Barki, H., & Hartwick, J. (2004). Conceptualizing the construct of interpersonal conflict. *The International Journal of Conflict Management, 15*(3), 216-244.
12	Personal integrity and sense of responsibility in effective leaders; egocentricism in university students. Required reading: Thomas, J. C. (2008). Ethical integrity in leadership and organizational moral culture. *Leadership, 4*(4), 419-442.
13	Self-leadership, mental health and effective leadership. Required reading: Dolbier, C. L., Soderstrom, M., & Steinhardt, M. A. (2001). The relationships between self-leadership and enhanced psychological, health and work outcomes. *Journal of Psychology, 135*, 469-485.

Table 3. Class schedule of the subject

Lecture	Content of Schedule
1	An overview of the subject and leadership concepts
2	Self-understanding
3	Emotional competence
4	Cognitive competence
5	Resilience
6	Spirituality
7	Ethics and morality
8	Social competence
9	Positive and healthy identity
10	Interpersonal communication
11	Group project presentation (Group 1 and Group 2); Interpersonal conflict, relationship building and team building
12	Group project presentation (Group 3 and Group 4); Integrity, sense of responsibility and egocentrism in university students
13	Group project presentation (Group 5 and Group 6); Self-leadership, mental health and effective leadership
14	Group project presentation (Group 7 and Group 8); Subject wrap up, review and evaluations

Similar to the pilot subject offered in 2010/11 academic year, several assessment methods were used to assess the performance of the students. These included class participation (20%), group project presentation (30%), and individual assignment (50%). To underscore the importance of student engagement, two forms of class participation were included. The first component was assessment by lecturers (15%), where student performance was assessed by class attendance (students are required to sign for class attendance), participation in class activities, pre-lecture preparation and completion of in-class and home assignments. The second component was assessment by group members (5%), where students were invited to evaluate the contribution and performance of each group member by completing a standardized form. The assessment methods and criteria for class participation can be seen in Table 4. Five scholarships funded by Wofoo Foundation with HK$5,000 each were awarded to five students with outstanding performance.

Table 4. Methods of assessment in the subject and criteria for participation

100% Continuous Assessment	Individual Assessment	Group Assessment
1. Class participation	20%	0%
2. Group project presentation	0%	30%
3. Term paper	50%	0%
Total	100%	

For the group project presentation, each presentation will last for 30 minutes. The medium of instruction and medium of assessment are in English.

Criteria of assessment for class participation (20%)

- *Assessment by Lecturer (15%):* Student performance is assessed by the following measures: a) class attendance (students are required to sign for class attendance); b) participation in class activities; c) preparation before class; and d) completion of in-class and take home tasks.
- *Assessment by Group Mates (5%):* Students will be invited to evaluate the contribution and performance of each group member by completing a standardized form. The Peer Assessment Form should be submitted to the lecturer together with the Group Presentation Declaration Form in a sealed envelope within one week after the group project presentation.

Table 5. Assignment of the subject (Group project presentation)

Group Project Presentation (30%):

Students are required to form groups to work on a project on **ONE chosen attribute of an effective leader** (e.g., emotional competence, moral competence). Only ONE attribute should be focused upon. It is expected that the group project will facilitate the development of the individual term paper. The group presentation will last for 30 minutes in the lecture.

Guidelines for Group Project Presentation

Students are required to choose an attribute of an effective leader based on the topics covered in the lectures. The attributes may include: positive and healthy identity, emotional competence, cognitive competence, resilience, spirituality, ethics and morality, social competence, conflict reolution skills. Students may also focus on topics not being covered in the subject after consulting the subject lecturer. Students will have to prepare the group presentation with reference to the following questions:

a) Review the conceptions and definitions of the chosen attribute;
b) Review one theory or model about the nature of the chosen attribute, such as factors affecting the development of the attribute (e.g., Kohlberg's theory on morality);
c) Present research findings and/or arguments from two studies showing the importance of this attribute (e.g., influence of spirituality on psychological well-being); and
d) Discuss two ways by which the chosen attribute can be strengthened for an individual.

It is expected that all members in the group will make equal contribution to the presentation. Students are required to complete a Group Presentation Declaration Form documenting the contribution of each of their group members.

Assessment Criteria for Group Presentation:

1. *Content*: Richness of the related knowledge in the presentation and thoroughness of the review (40%)
2. *Higher-level thinking:* Depth of discussion on the theoretical issues; level of critical discussion; integration of the theories and research findings reviewed; level of reflection (40%)
3. *Quality of the presentation:* Flow of arguments, division of labor, ability to engage the classmates, ability to complete the presentation within the allocated time (20%)

Consistent with the first piloting exercise, there were two assignments for the students. The first one was the group project presentation (30%). Students were required to form groups to work on a project on one chosen attribute of an effective leader based on the topics covered in the lectures (e.g., resilience, emotional competence, moral competence, etc.). The detailed requirements can be seen in Table 5. Besides the group project presentation, students were required to write a term paper with two parts (at least 1,500 words excluding references). The details can be seen in Table 6. The rubrics for marking with specific reference to outstanding and exceptionally outstanding papers can be seen in Table 7. Finally, a relevant and comprehensive reading list was developed for the student (Table 8). The Peer Assessment Form and the Group Presentation Declaration Form can be seen in Appendix 1 and Appendix 2, respectively.

Table 6. Assignment of the subject (Individual term paper)

Term Paper (50%):

Students are required to write a term paper with two parts (at least 1,500 words excluding references). In the first part, students are required to *critically discuss the concepts of leadership quality covered in the group presentation* on the conceptual level (around 750 words). In the second part, students are expected to *evaluate the extent to which you possess this leadership quality* based on a thorough reflection of your life experiences (around 750 words). The term paper accounts for 50% of the final grade. The term paper should be submitted within one week after the last session (the exact submission date will be announced by the lecturer).

Each student will receive a class ID and an enrollment password of TURNITIN system (i.e., a system checking for plagiarism) by email about one month before the assignment deadline. You are required to follow the steps of the Turnitin Student Quickstart to check your assignments and print out the Originality Report. You should submit a hard copy of your assignment together with the Originality Report to your lecturer. Your term paper will not be marked if the Originality

Report is not attached.

Assessment Criteria for the Term Paper

Part 1

- *Content:* Richness of the related knowledge in the paper; evidence of extensive and extra readings (40%)
- *Higher-level thinking:* Depth of discussion on the theoretical issues; level of critical discussion; integration of the theories and research findings reviewed; level of reflection (40%)
- *Quality of the paper:* Flow of arguments; clarity; use of English; typographical errors; correct references format (e.g., APA style) (20%)

Part 2

- *Content:* Richness of the reflection, presentation and analysis; evidence presented in relation to the problem; degree of passion (30%)
- *Higher-level thinking:* Integration of concepts and personal life; arguments supporting conclusions; level of reflection; insights based on self-examination (50%)
- *Quality of the paper*: Flow of arguments; clarity; use of English; typographical errors; correct references format (APA style) (20%)

Table 7. Attributes of an outstanding /exceptionally outstanding group presentation and individual paper

Attributes of an Outstanding/Exceptionally Outstanding Group Presentation:

- Content: Concepts and ideas are discussed clearly and thoroughly; provide an extensive presentation with a variety of primary and secondary sources to support the topic; evidence of clear thoughts and easy to follow the line of reasoning; demonstrate a clear and in-depth understanding of the relevant topics; cited materials are well integrated; literature review is very extensive.
- Higher-level Thinking: Discuss views from different perspectives and show deep personal understanding of theories and findings; critically reflect upon one's own assertions and refute bias; effectively synthesize theory and research findings with personal experience; able to raise and analyze thought-provoking questions and help audience gain insights; use reasonable judgment and make convincing and rational conclusion.
- Quality of Presentation: Ideas and topics are presented not only clearly but in an interesting and unique way; use grammar and vocabulary accurately; excellent work distribution and show great collaboration among group members; appropriate length of presentation; actively engage the audience; complete on time with appropriate time allocation for each session.

Attributes of an Outstanding/ Exceptionally Outstanding Paper (Part 1):

- Content: Concepts and ideas are presented clearly; very rich content; shows extensive research with a variety of primary and secondary sources to support the topic; quotations are effectively used to guide reader; has a thorough understanding of the topic; demonstrates a clear and in-depth understanding of the relevant topics; maintains a clear focus on the topic; cited materials are well integrated.
- Higher-Order Thinking: Extensive discussion of views from different perspectives; shows a deep personal understanding of theories and findings; critically reflects upon one's own assertions and refutes bias; effectively synthesizes theories and research findings with personal experience; able to raise and analyze thought-provoking questions and help readers gain insights; use reasonable judgment and make convincing and rational conclusion.
- Quality of the Paper: Absence of punctuation, spelling and writing errors; paper is well organized and coherently developed; ideas and topics are supported by compelling evidence and argumentation; evidence of clear thoughts and easy to follow the line of reasoning; using APA format correctly and consistently; all references are included in the reference list.

Attributes of an Outstanding/ Exceptionally Outstanding Paper (Part 2):

- Content: Demonstrates an in-depth self-understanding; shows very detailed self-disclosure of views, feelings and thoughts; using a variety of personal experiences and appropriate examples to support the topic; maintains a clear focus on the topic; cited materials are well integrated in sentences.
- Higher-Order Thinking: Ideas are supported by compelling evidence and arguments; critically reflect upon one's own assertions and refute bias; effectively synthesize theories and research findings with personal experience; clearly displays novelty and originality; able to raise and analyze thought-provoking questions and help audience gain insights; demonstrates insight and its significance through self-awareness and learning.
- Quality of the Paper: Absence of punctuation, spelling and writing errors; paper is well organized and coherently developed; ideas and topics are supported by compelling evidence and arguments; evidence of clear thoughts and easy to follow the line of reasoning; using APA format correctly and consistently; all references are included in the reference list.

Table 8. Reading lists of the subject

Adair, J. E. (2005). How to grow leaders: *The seven key principles of effective leadership development.* USA: Kogan Page.

Burke, R. J., & Cooper, C. L. (Eds.). (2006). *Inspiring leaders.* New York: Routledge.

Cangemi, J. P., Burga, B., Lazarus, H., Miller, R. L., & Fitzgerald, J. (2008). The real work of the leader: A focus on the human side of the equation. *Journal of Management Development, 27*(10), 1026-1036.

Hannah, S. T., Woolfolk, R. L., & Lord, R. G. (2009). Leader self-structure: A framework for positive leadership. *Journal of Organizational Behavior, 30*(2), 269-290.

Hogan, R., & Kaiser, R. B. (2005). What we know about leadership. *Review of General Psychology, 9*(2), 169-180.

Knapp, M. L., & Daly, J. A. (Eds.). (2002). *Handbook of interpersonal communication* (3rd ed.). CA: Sage Publications.

Komives, S. R., Lucas, N., & McMahon, T. R. (2007). *Exploring leadership: For college students who want to make a difference.* San Francisco, CA: Jossey-Bass.

London, M. (2002). *Leadership development: Paths to self-insight and professional growth.* Mahwah, NJ: Lawrence Erlbaum Associates.

Roberts, D. C. (2007). *Deeper learning in leadership: Helping college students find the potential within.* San Francisco, CA: Jossey-Bass.

Shek, D. T. L. (2010). Nurturing holistic development of university students in Hong Kong: Where are we and where should we go? *Scientific World Journal, 10*, 563-575.

Shek, D. T. L., Ma, H. K., & Merrick, J. (Eds.). (2007). Positive youth development: Development of a pioneering program in a Chinese context. London: Freund.

Shek, D. T. L., & Wong, K. K. (2011). Do adolescent developmental issues disappear overnight? Reflections about holistic development in university students. *ScientificWorldJOURNAL, 10*, 353-361.

van Knippenberg, D., van Knippenberg, B., de Cremer, D., & Hogg, M. A. (2004). Leadership, self, and identity: A review and research agenda. *The Leadership Quarterly, 15*, 825-856.

Wood, J. T. (2004). *Interpersonal communication: Everyday encounters* (4th ed.). Belmont, CA: Thomson/Wadsworth.

Supplementary references

Antonakis, J., Ashkanasy, N. M., & Dasborough, M. T. (2009). Does leadership need emotional intelligence? *The Leadership Quarterly, 20*(2), 247-261.

Avolio, B. J. (2007). Promoting more integrative strategies for leadership theory-building. *American Psychologist, 62*(1), 25-33.

Burke, R. J. (2006). Why leaders fail: Exploring the darkside. *International Journal of Manpower, 27*(1), 91-100.

Fry, L. W. (2003). Toward a theory of spiritual leadership. *The Leadership Quarterly, 14*, 693-727.

Humphrey, J. H. (2003). *Stress education for college students*. New York: Novinka Books.

Lin, C. (2008). Demystifying the chameleonic nature of Chinese leadership. *Journal of Leadership and Organizational Studies, 14*(4), 303-321.

Lord, R. G., & Brown, D. J. (2004). *Leadership processes and follower self-identity*. Mahwah, NJ: Lawrence Erlbaum Associates.

Messick, D. M., & Kramer, R. M. (2005). *The psychology of leadership: New perspectives and research*. Mahwah, NJ: Lawrence Erlbaum Associates.

Runde, C. E., & Flanagan, T. A. (2007). *Becoming a conflict competent leader: How you and your organization can manage conflict effectively*. San Francisco, CA: Jossey-Bass.

Shankman, M. L., & Allen, S. J. (2008). *Emotionally intelligent leadership: A guide for college students*. San Francisco, CA: Jossey-Bass.

Topchik, G. S. (2007). *The first-time manager's guide to team building*. New York: AMACOM.

EVALUATION STRATEGIES AND PRELIMINARY EVALUATION FINDINGS

In the first piloting exercise, several evaluation studies were conducted (1-7). First, adopting a prestest-posttest pre-experimental design, objective outcome evaluation findings revealed that students showed improvement in measures of holistic development and psychosocial competencies after taking the subject. Second, subjective outcome evaluation findings collected after each lecture and at the end of the course showed that students had positive evaluation of the subject, lecturers as well as perceived benefits of the subject. Third, systematic class observations (i.e., process evaluation) showed that there was high program adherence and students generally had good participation and responses in class. Fourth, qualitative evaluation based on reflective notes written by the students showed that students generally had positive perceptions of the subject and the benefits of the program. Fifth, from the writings of the scholarship recipients of the subject, it was found that the subject could benefit the students. Finally, qualitative findings based on focus groups showed that students had positive evaluation of the subject, although some recommendations were also made.

In the second piloting exercise, several evaluation strategies were used. First, besides collecting pretest and posttest data from the students taking this subject, data were also collected from students of a control group. Second, post-lecture evaluation data were collected. Third, subjective outcome evaluation data based on post-lecture assessment were collected. Fourth, process evaluation based on systematic observations was carried out. Fifth, qualitative data based on reflective notes completed by the students were collected. Sixth, qualitative data collected via focus groups were analyzed. Finally, reflections written by students were collected in this study. Preliminary analyses of the evaluation data analyzed so far revealed the following observations:

- *Post-Course Subjective Outcome Evaluation:* The quantitative findings presented in the chapter in this special issue generally showed that the students had positive evaluation of the content of the course and the lecturers. Furthermore, students generally perceived the course to be beneficial to their development. Actually, the post-course evaluation findings were more favourable than those reported in the first piloting exercise.
- *Post-Lecture Subjective Outcome Evaluation:* Based on the quantitative evaluation findings presented in the chapter in this special issue, it was found that the students had positive evaluation of the content of the lecture and the lecturers. Furthermore, students generally perceived the lectures to be beneficial to their development. Actually, the post-lecture evaluation findings were more favourable than those reported in the first piloting exercise.
- *Process Evaluation:* Based on systematic observations of 9 lectures by two independent observers, process evaluation findings showed that program adherence was high and the program implementation quality was high.
- *Qualitative Evaluation (Reflection):* Based on 104 pieces of reflections collected from students, analyses showed that students had positive evaluation of the subject, class and lecturers and they perceived that there were benefits of the subject.

DISCUSSION

This chapter outlines the characteristics of a credit-bearing course entitled "Tomorrow's Leaders" at The Hong Kong Polytechnic University. Several observations can be highlighted from the preliminary evaluation findings. First, the students generally had positive evaluation of the subject. Second, teachers were seen in a very favourable manner by the students. Third, students generally perceived that the subject was beneficial to their development. Fourth, the subject and related evaluation findings are consistent with the findings of the previous validation exercise. Finally, the tentative findings are consistent with the findings in the positive youth development literature that positive youth development programs are beneficial to adolescent development (8-15). As there are few related programs in the literature, this is an important addition to the literature.

ACKNOWLEDGMENTS

The development of the course titled "Tomorrow's Leaders" and the evaluation study were financially supported by The Hong Kong Polytechnic University via the Teaching Development Grant and the funding for the 3-3-4 new curriculum. We would also like to thank the Wofoo Foundation for the establishment of several scholarships for those outstanding students taking the course. This chapter has been published as a paper in the

International Journal on Disability and Human Development, 2013;12(2). Permission has been obtained from De Gruyter to re-publish in this modified form.

APPENDIX 1: PEER ASSESSMENT FORM

THE HONG KONG POLYTECHNIC UNIVERSITY
DEPARTMENT OF APPLIED SOCIAL SCIENCES
APSS2816 TOMORROW'S LEADERS

PEER ASSESSMENT FORM

Dear ______________________ (Name of Assessor),

To assess class participation, please give a mark to each group member (ranging from "0" to "5" marks) which best describes his/her performance and contribution in your group. You are not required to assess your own performance in the group. Your assessment will contribute to the final subject grade of your group mates (5% of the total marks).

Name of the Group ______________________________

Name of Your Group Members	Marks (0 -5)
1.	
2.	
3.	
4.	
5.	
6.	
7.	
8.	
9.	
10.	

____

Signature Date

APPENDIX 2: GROUP PRESENTATION DECLARATION FORM

THE HONG KONG POLYTECHNIC UNIVERSITY
DEPARTMENT OF APPLIED SOCIAL SCIENCES
APSS2816 TOMORROW'S LEADERS

Group Presentation Declaration Form

Name of the Group: _____________

We hereby declare that the work done for the group presentation and the presentation outline/material is equally / not equally* shared among the group members. With reference to the work done (i.e., 100%), the contribution of individual members is as follows:

Member 1:
Name: _____________
Contribution: % of the total work done
Signature:
Date:

Member 2:
Name: _____________
Contribution: % of the total work done
Signature:
Date:

Member 3:
Name: _____________
Contribution: % of the total work done
Signature:
Date:

Member 4:
Name: _____________
Contribution: % of the total work done
Signature:
Date:

Member 5:
Name: _____________
Contribution: % of the total work done
Signature:
Date:

Member 6:
Name: _____________
Contribution: % of the total work done
Signature:
Date:

Member 7:
Name: _____________
Contribution: % of the total work done
Signature:
Date:

Member 8:
Name: _____________
Contribution: % of the total work done
Signature:
Date:

Member 9:
Name: _____________
Contribution: % of the total work done
Signature:
Date:

Member 10:
Name: _____________
Contribution: % of the total work done
Signature:
Date:

* Delete whichever not applicable.

REFERENCES

[1] Shek DTL, Sun RCF. Promoting psychosocial competencies in university students: evaluation based on a one group pretest-posttest design. Int J Disabil Hum Dev 2012;11:229-34.

[2] Shek DTL, Sun RCF. Promoting leadership and intrapersonal competence in university students: what can we learn from Hong Kong? Int J Disabil Hum Dev 2012;11:221-8.

[3] Shek DTL, Sun RCF. Process evaluation of a positive youth development course in a university setting in Hong Kong. Int J Disabil Hum Dev 2012;11:235-41.

[4] Shek DTL, Sun RCF. Qualitative evaluation of a positive youth development course in a university setting in Hong Kong. Int J Disabil Hum Dev 2012;11:243-8.

[5] Shek DTL, Sun RCF. Focus group evaluation of a positive youth development course in a university in Hong Kong. Int J Disabil Hum Dev 2012;11:249-54.

[6] Shek DTL. Post-lecture evaluation of a positive youth development subject for university students in Hong Kong. Int J Disabil Hum Dev 2013, 7 pages. DOI: 10.1515/ijdhd-2013-0011.

[7] Shek DTL, Wu FKY. Reflective journals of students taking a positive youth development course in a university context in Hong Kong. ScientificWorldJournal, 2012, Article ID 131560, 8 pages. DOI: 10.1100/2012/131560.

[8] Shek DTL, Ma CMS, Tang CYP. Predictors of subjective outcome evaluation findings in a positive youth development program in Hong Kong. Int J Disabil Hum Dev 2011;10:249-55.

[9] Shek DTL, Sun RCF, Merrick J. Training programs and implementation process of positive youth development programs. Int J Adolesc Med Health 2011;23:303-4.

[10] Shek DTL, Ma HK, Sun RCF. A brief overview of adolescent developmental problems in Hong Kong. ScientificWorldJournal 2011;11:2243-56.

[11] Shek DTL, Ma HK, Sun RCF. Development of a new curriculum in a positive youth development program: the Project P.A.T.H.S. in Hong Kong ScientificWorldJournal 2011;11:2207-18.

[12] Shek DTL. Quality of life research: responses to emerging issues in a changing world. Soc Indic Res 2011;100:371-4.

[13] Shek DTL. Subjective outcome and objective outcome evaluation findings: insights from a Chinese context. Res Social Work Pract 2010;20:293-301.

[14] Sun RCF, Shek DTL. Positive youth development, life satisfaction and problem behaviour among Chinese adolescents in Hong Kong: a replication. Soc Indic Res 2012;105:541-59.

[15] Shek DTL, Yu L. Longitudinal impact of the Project P.A.T.H.S. on adolescent risk behavior: what happened after five years? ScientificWorldJournal 2012, Article ID 316029, 13 pages. DOI:10.1100/2012/316029.

In: Chinese Adolescent Development ISBN: 978-1-62618-622-4
Editors: Daniel TL Shek, Rachel CF Sun, Joav Merrick © 2013 Nova Science Publishers, Inc.

Chapter 8

POST-LECTURE EVALUATION OF A UNIVERSITY COURSE ON LEADERSHIP AND INTRAPERSONAL DEVELOPMENT

Daniel TL Shek *[*,1,2,3,4,5]*
and Rachel CF Sun *[6]*
[1]Department of Applied Social Sciences,
The Hong Kong Polytechnic University, Hong Kong, PRC
[2]Centre for Innovative Programmes for Adolescents and Families,
The Hong Kong Polytechnic University, Hong Kong, PRC
[3]Kiang Wu Nursing College of Macau, Macau, PRC
[4]Department of Social Work,
East China Normal University, Shanghai, PRC
[5]Division of Adolescent Medicine, Department of Pediatrics,
Kentucky Children's Hospital, University of Kentucky College of Medicine,
Lexington, Kentucky, US
[6]Faculty of Education, The University of Hong Kong,
Hong Kong, PRC

ABSTRACT

Post-lecture evaluation findings of a subject on leadership and intrapersonal development designed to promote holistic development of university students at The Hong Kong Polytechnic University in Hong Kong were reported. In the first 13 lectures, students were invited to respond to a 12-item post-lecture questionnaire after each lecture. Normative findings showed that students generally had positive perceptions of the subject, class and teacher attributes, and the overall evaluation was very positive. Factor analyses showed that three factors were abstracted from the scale, including Subject Attributes,

[*] Correspondence: Professor Daniel TL Shek, PhD, FHKPS, BBS, JP, Chair Professor of Applied Social Sciences, Faculty of Health and Social Sciences, Department of Applied Social Sciences, The Hong Kong Polytechnic University, Room HJ407, Core H, Hunghom, Hong Kong. E-mail: daniel.shek@polyu.edu.hk

Class Attributes and Teacher Attributes. The total scale and subscales were internally consistent. Regarding predictors of global evaluation of the subject and the teacher, multiple regression analyses showed that subject, class and teacher attributes were significant predictors.

INTRODUCTION

There are views suggesting that there are worrying trends in the development of university students in Hong Kong. Shek (1) pointed out that four developmental issues deserved our attention. First, university students did not have a high level of civic engagement and they were relatively politically apathetic. Second, research findings revealed that there were mental health problems among university students. Third, evidence showed that employers in Hong Kong were not satisfied with the attributes of graduates (such as interpersonal cooperation and maturity); and finally, personal qualities of local university graduates were seen as worse than those in mainland China.

There are other research findings showing that the development of university students in Hong Kong deserving our attention. For example, Tsui and Wing (2) reported that the actual sleep duration among students was far less than their expected sleep duration, with roughly 72% of the participants could be regarded as having sleep deprivation. Sing and Wong (3) further reported that insomnia was identified as a prevalent problem in university students, with 68.6% of the sample classified as insomniacs. Besides, levels of drinking, binge drinking, and alcohol abuse for Year 2 students were significantly higher than those of freshmen (4). Research also revealed that roughly 15% of university students could be classified as heavy Internet users with 4 or more hours per day (5). In addition to problems in lifestyle and health behavior, research also showed that university students were reluctant to challenge experts and they lacked confidence to deal conflict (6). In a study of the prevalence of physical assault against dating partners in university students in Hong Kong, Chan et al. (7) showed that physical assault in the preceding year was 46% which was higher than those reported in the International Dating Violence study.

As pointed out by Shek (8), adolescent developmental issues simply do not disappear over-night when high school students enter universities. Therefore, it is important for youth researchers and workers to examine how holistic development in university students could possibly be promoted. While developmental issues in university students are commonly handled by student affairs offices where clinical counseling models are usually adopted, such approach is remedial in nature and the coverage of issues in university students is narrow. Based on the public health approach, it is argued that it is more effective to have universal prevention programs than simply providing remedial services. With reference to the positive youth development approach, cultivating of psychosocial competencies in young people represents a promising approach to promote holistic development in university students. Actually, positive youth development constructs have been widely used in curricula-based programs to promote holistic development of students in high school contexts. For example, Catalano et al. (9) identified 15 positive youth development constructs in the available successful programs. These include: bonding, resilience, psychosocial competencies (cognitive, emotional, social, behavioral and moral competencies), self-determination, self-efficacy, clear and positive identity, spirituality, beliefs in the future, prosocial norms, prosocial involvement and recognition for positive behavior.

Under the new 4-year curriculum in The Hong Kong Polytechnic University, there is a requirement in the area of "Leadership and Intrapersonal Development". With specific reference to this requirement, a subject entitled "Tomorrow's Leaders" was developed by the authors based on the positive youth development framework. The positive youth development constructs covered in the course included self-understanding, emotional competence, cognitive competence, resilience, spirituality, social competence, moral competence, positive identity, interpersonal communication, conflict resolution, personal integrity, self-leadership and self-reflection. Through lectures, class activities and assignments, students are helped to understand the attributes of a successful leader, conduct personal reflections and cultivate their awareness of the importance of intrapersonal and interpersonal attributes of university students. Conceptually speaking, the topics covered in the course are based on the positive youth development framework which is also adopted in the Project P.A.T.H.S. in Hong Kong, with has been consistently shown to be able to promote holistic development in junior secondary school students in Hong Kong (10-14).

The subject "Tomorrow's Leaders" was piloted in 2010-11 school year. To triangulate the evaluation findings, different evaluation strategies were used (15-24). First, utilizing a one-group pretest-posttest design, pretest and posttest data were collected from the students taking the course to reveal changes in the students based on objective outcome measures. Second, post-course subjective outcome evaluation was carried out where a questionnaire covering measures of the course, instructor and perceived effectiveness of the course program was distributed to the students in the last lecture. Third, post-lecture evaluation for the first 13 lectures was carried out. Fourth, through systematic observations, process evaluation was conducted by two trained colleagues to understand the program implementation details in 14 lectures as well as program adherence. Fifth, qualitative evaluation using focus groups and reflection notes were conducted. Overall speaking, different evaluation findings strongly suggest that the subject was able to promote holistic development in the students taking this subject.

To further test out the subject, "Tomorrow's Leaders" was piloted again in the first term of 2011/12 school year. Consistent with the first piloting exercise, multiple evaluation strategies were used to examine the effectiveness of the subject. In this chapter, evaluation findings based on post-lecture evaluation are presented. There are several arguments for conducting post-lecture evaluation. First, in contrast to post-course subjective outcome evaluation which yields relatively global information (e.g., degree of interaction in class), detailed information about the relevance of the lecture content and quality of lecture delivery can be revealed by post-lecture evaluation. Such specific information is very important as far as lecture development and refinement is concerned. Second, post-lecture evaluation can yield immediate information that can be used by the instructor to plan for the next lecture. This is in sharp contrast to post-course evaluation where the timeliness of evaluation findings may not be good. Finally, while general impression of the students is gauged in post-course evaluation, specific perceptions of a particular lecture can be assessed in post-lecture evaluation. The fresh memory in connection with post-lecture evaluation may also yield more meaningful and valid subjective outcome evaluation data.

There are several purposes of the present study. First, profiles of responses of the students to the post-lecture evaluation questionnaire were presented. Second, dimensionality of the scale assessing post-lecture evaluation was investigated. Third, reliability of the total scale and the subscales were examined. Finally, predictors of global evaluation of the subject and the teacher were investigated.

OUR STUDY

In the second piloting exercise, the subject was offered to four classes of students, with a total of 195 students (49 in Class A, 48 in Class B, 49 in Class C and 49 in Class D). At the end of Lecture 1 to Lecture 13, students were invited to respond to a subjective outcome evaluation form regarding the content and process of the lecture and the teacher. There are 12 items and one open-ended question in the evaluation form. The items cover different topics including design, atmosphere, peer interaction, student interest, student participation, opportunities for reflection, degree of helpfulness to personal development, instructor's mastery of lecture, instructor's use of teaching methods, whether knowledge helpful to students, global evaluation of lecture, and global evaluation of the lecturer. The respondents were required to respond on a six-point scales with "Strongly Disagree", "Disagree", "Slightly Disagree", "Slightly Agree", "Agree", and "Strongly Agree". The items are as follows:

- Item 1: The design of this lecture was very good.
- Item 2: The classroom atmosphere of this lecture was very pleasant.
- Item 3: There was much peer interaction amongst the students in this lecture.
- Item 4: I am interested in the content of this lecture.
- Item 5: There was much student participation in this lecture.
- Item 6: There were many opportunities for reflection in this lecture.
- Item 7: This lecture is helpful to my personal development.
- Item 8: The lecturer had a good mastery of the lecture material.
- Item 9: The lecturer used different methods to encourage students to learn.
- Item 10: The lecturer in this lecture was able to help students understand the knowledge covered in the lecture.
- Item 11: Overall speaking, I have very positive evaluation of the lecturer in this lecture
- Item 12: Overall speaking, I have very positive evaluation of this lecture.

Conceptually speaking, it was hypothesized that items 1, 4, 6 and 7 are related to the attributes of the subject (Subject Attributes), items 2, 3 and 5 are related to the attributes of the class (Class Attributes), and items 8, 9 and 10 were related to the attributes of the teacher (Teacher Attributes). Item 11 and Item 12 are items that are designed to assess the global evaluation of the teacher and the course.

A total of 2,012 questionnaires were collected for all lectures throughout the course. On the day of data collection, the purpose of the evaluation was mentioned, and confidentiality of the data was repeatedly emphasized to all students. All participants responded to the items and question in the evaluation form in a self-administration format. Adequate time was provided for the participants to complete the questionnaire. In the present chapter, focus would be put on the findings based on the quantitative data.

Data analysis

Descriptive statistical analyses were used to examine the perceptions of the students on the course and teacher performance. Factor analysis was performed for the Lecture 1 data (i.e., first batch of data to avoid non-independence of observations) to examine the structure of Item 1 to Item 10 to see whether there was supported for the three dimensions – subject attributes, class attributes and teacher attributes. To enlarge the sample size, the sample in Study 1 was also included for analysis. To examine whether subject attributes, class attributes and teacher attributes predicted the overall evaluation of the teacher (Item 11) and the subject (Item 12), multiple regression analyses were performed. All analyses were performed by using the Statistical Package for Social Sciences Version 16.0.

FINDINGS

A total of 2,012 post-lecture subjective outcome evaluation forms were collected after Lecture 1 to Lecture 13. As findings based on the closed-ended questions are presented in this chapter, descriptive findings based on percentages and means are presented in Table 1 and Table 2, respectively. Several observations can be highlighted from the percentage findings presented in Table 1. In the first place, most participants generally had positive perceptions of the course. For example, 92.7% of the participants regarded the program design as positive; 89.6% of the participants agreed that class promoted reflection. Besides, students perceived the class atmosphere to be pleasant (item 2: 91%), with much peer interaction (item 3: 90.3%) and student participation (item 5: 90.2%). Finally, teachers were perceived to have good mastery of the course (item 8), use varied teaching methods (item 9) and to be able to help students understand knowledge (item 10). Regarding global evaluation of the subject, 94.4% and 92.6% had positive evaluation of the teacher and subject, respectively.

As different dimensions of the scale were expected to be inter-correlated, factor analysis with non-orthogonal rotation was used. Combining the data in Study 1 and Study 2, principal factor analysis followed by Promax rotation showed that three factors could be meaningfully extracted, accounting for 60.49% of the variance.

Factor I included items 1, 4, 6 and 7 and it was labeled a Subject Attributes factor (alpha = .84, mean inter-item correlation = .57). The second factor included items 2, 3 and 5 (alpha = .82, mean inter-item correlation = .61). Because these items are basically concerned with lecture delivery in class, this factor was labeled Class Attributes factor. The third factor included items 8, 9 and 10 that could be labeled a Teacher Attributes factor (alpha = .80; mean inter-item correlation = .58). The pattern matrix can be seen in Table 3.

Further analyses showed that the factor structure of the scale was moderately consistent across Study 1 and Study 2 (coefficients of congruence =.74, .85 and .75 for Subject Attributes, Class Attributes and Teacher Attributes, respectively). The total scale was also found to be internally consistent ((alpha = .93, mean inter-item correlation = .52).

Table 1. Mean ratings by the students from lecture 1 to lecture 13

	Lecture													
Item	**L1**	**L2**	**L3**	**L4**	**L5**	**L6**	**L7**	**L8**	**L9**	**L10**	**L11**	**L12**	**L13**	**Mean**
1. Good lecture design	4.57	4.54	4.48	4.40	4.75	4.57	4.53	4.59	4.65	4.86	4.43	4.52	4.49	**4.57**
2. Atmosphere was very good	4.70	4.61	4.58	4.38	4.72	4.40	4.58	4.59	4.79	4.84	4.44	4.41	4.34	**4.57**
3. Much peer interaction	4.59	4.81	4.78	4.50	4.76	4.42	4.63	4.68	4.80	4.96	4.33	4.28	4.25	**4.60**
4. Interested in the content	4.55	4.61	4.43	4.37	4.80	4.51	4.51	4.72	4.74	4.82	4.43	4.52	4.49	**4.58**
5. Much student participation	4.52	4.69	4.67	4.43	4.76	4.36	4.52	4.58	4.81	4.92	4.40	4.30	4.23	**4.55**
6. Many opportunities for reflection	4.59	4.54	4.42	4.32	4.80	4.69	4.50	4.59	4.74	4.71	4.43	4.48	4.46	**4.56**
7. Helpful to my personal development	4.57	4.57	4.52	4.33	4.91	4.64	4.55	4.66	4.77	4.78	4.52	4.57	4.44	**4.60**
8. Lecturer had good mastery of lecture	4.86	4.69	4.53	4.41	4.83	4.62	4.61	4.75	4.70	4.84	4.53	4.63	4.56	**4.66**
9. Varied teaching methods used	4.73	4.68	4.56	4.54	4.73	4.59	4.68	4.66	4.72	4.95	4.55	4.51	4.49	**4.65**
10. Helpful to students (knowledge)	4.56	4.69	4.55	4.45	4.71	4.55	4.64	4.71	4.66	4.79	4.59	4.58	4.51	**4.61**
11. Very positive evaluation of the lecturer	4.81	4.78	4.62	4.48	4.83	4.66	4.70	4.74	4.73	4.89	4.44	4.59	4.55	**4.68**
12. Very positive evaluation of the lecture	4.63	4.61	4.53	4.41	4.74	4.55	4.60	4.68	4.76	4.91	4.48	4.55	4.43	**4.61**
Number of questionnaires collected	**176**	**173**	**165**	**168**	**143**	**166**	**152**	**152**	**129**	**116**	**162**	**155**	**155**	**2012**

Table 2. Percentage findings based on subjective outcome evaluation of each lecture

Item	Percentage of positive responses for different lectures													
	1	**2**	**3**	**4**	**5**	**6**	**7**	**8**	**9**	**10**	**11**	**12**	**13**	**Overall**
1. Good lecture design	97.2	93.6	90.9	89.3	97.2	91.6	90.1	91.4	95.3	96.6	90.1	93.5	89.7	92.7
2. Atmosphere was very good	94.3	92.4	93.3	84.5	95.8	86.7	90.1	91.4	96.9	92.2	89.5	90.3	87.1	91.0
3. Much peer interaction	92.6	93.6	94.5	89.3	95.8	85.5	90.1	94.1	99.2	94.8	85.8	83.2	77.9	90.3
4. Interested in the content	94.3	93.6	86.1	85.7	97.2	87.3	88.0	92.1	96.1	94.8	88.9	89.7	89.0	90.8
5. Much student participation	89.8	94.8	92.7	89.3	93.7	86.7	89.5	93.4	95.3	95.7	89.5	85.2	79.9	90.2
6. Many opportunities for reflection	88.6	87.9	87.3	83.3	95.1	91.6	87.5	93.4	95.3	93.9	87.0	89.7	87.7	89.6
7. Helpful to my personal development	92.6	91.3	90.9	89.3	97.2	92.2	92.1	94.1	96.1	93.9	91.4	93.5	88.3	92.4
8. Lecturer had good mastery of lecture	96.6	91.9	90.3	87.5	95.8	91.0	89.5	95.4	96.9	95.7	94.4	93.5	92.9	93.0
9. Varied teaching methods used	94.3	91.9	91.5	90.5	97.2	92.2	92.8	94.1	96.9	96.5	94.4	88.4	89.5	92.9
10. Helpful to students (knowledge)	92.0	95.3	92.7	88.1	97.2	92.2	88.8	94.7	93.8	92.2	94.4	94.8	91.5	92.9
11. Very positive evaluation of the lecturer	96.0	96.5	93.3	91.7	97.2	92.2	94.1	96.1	97.7	98.3	89.5	94.8	92.2	94.4
12. Very positive evaluation of the lecture	94.3	93.6	92.1	88.7	97.2	89.2	90.8	93.4	97.7	94.0	91.4	92.9	90.9	92.6
Coefficient alpha for the 12-item scale	.92	.95	.95	.96	.93	.96	.96	.95	.95	.95	.96	.95	.95	.95
Mean inter-item correlation	.50	.61	.64	.68	.52	.67	.65	.64	.61	.63	.68	.63	.62	.63
Number of questionnaires collected	**176**	**173**	**165**	**168**	**143**	**166**	**152**	**152**	**129**	**116**	**162**	**155**	**155**	**2012**

Note: The cumulative percentage based on "Strongly Agree", "Agree" and "Slightly Agree" for an item is presented for each lecture.

Table 3. Dimensionality of the post-lecture evaluation scale in Study 1, Study 2 and the combined sample

Item	Study 1			Study 2			Total		
	F1	F2	F3	F1	F2	F3	F1	F2	F3
1. The design of this lecture was very good.	**0.429**	0.375	0.079	0.100	0.000	**0.665**	**0.397**	0.264	0.181
2. The classroom atmosphere of this lecture was very pleasant.	-0.010	**0.798**	0.090	-0.059	**0.447**	0.349	0.016	**0.673**	0.147
3. There was much peer interaction amongst the students in this lecture.	-0.1081	**0.925**	-0.051	-0.077	**0.930**	-0.078	-0.074	**0.921**	-0.086
4. I am interested in the content of this lecture.	**0.662**	0.168	0.018	-0.079	-0.070	**0.907**	**0.648**	0.141	0.026
5. There was much student participation in this lecture.	0.154	**0.557**	0.138	0.089	**0.681**	-0.022	0.111	**0.633**	0.056
6. There were many opportunities for reflection in this lecture.	**0.792**	-0.179	0.113	**0.482**	0.246	0.037	**0.669**	-0.104	0.139
7. This lecture is helpful to my personal development.	**0.868**	0.010	-0.121	0.232	0.044	**0.551**	**0.943**	-0.010	-0.139
8. The lecturer had a good mastery of the lecture material.	0.150	0.004	**0.651**	**0.301**	0.229	0.264	0.169	0.076	**0.555**
9. The lecturer used different methods to encourage students to learn.	-0.170	0.098	**0.864**	**0.512**	0.137	0.074	-0.169	0.083	**0.857**
10. The lecturer in this lecture was able to help students understand the knowledge covered in the lecture.	0.179	-0.032	**0.669**	**1.010**	-0.155	-0.040	0.232	-0.118	**0.680**
Eigen Value	5.69	1.01	0.77	5.16	0.99	0.75	5.41	1.00	0.78
Variance Explained	53.29	6.47	4.15	47.34	6.39	3.52	50.17	6.25	4.07

Study 1: F1= Subject Attributes factor. F2 = Class Attributes factor. F3 = Teacher Attributes factor.
Study 2: F1= Teacher Attributes factor. F2 = Class Attributes factor. F3 = Subject Attributes factor.
Combined: F1= Subject Attributes factor. F2 = Class Attributes factor. F3 = Teacher Attributes factor.

Table 4. Predictors of global evaluation of the teacher and global evaluation of the lecture

Analyses	Lecture													
	1	**2**	**3**	**4**	**5**	**6**	**7**	**8**	**9**	**10**	**11**	**12**	**13**	**Overall**
DV: Global Perception of the Teacher (Item 11): Predictors														
Subject Attribute	.32***	.32***	.33***	.43***	.28***	.42***	.37***	.25**	.41***	.05	.28*	.31**	.22**	.31***
Class Attribute	.14*	.20**	.27***	-.03	.29**	.09	.12	.34***	.01	.14	.27**	.13	.09	.16***
Teacher Attribute	.42***	.37***	.33***	.49***	.34***	.44***	.42***	.27**	.46***	.65***	.32**	.41***	.60***	.42***
R Square	.61	.65	.73	.74	.63	.79	.74	.65	.67	.64	.66	.64	.73	.69
DV: Global Perception of the Course (Item 12): Predictors														
Subject Attribute	.40***	.44***	.41***	.45***	.44***	.47***	.28**	.30**	.33***	.34**	.42***	.32***	.64***	.41***
Class Attribute	.27***	.32***	.20**	.08	.14	.23**	.15*	.31**	.19	.12	.26**	.14	.10	.20***
Teacher Attribute	.24***	.17**	.33***	.39***	.25**	.25***	.49***	.25*	.39***	.44***	.22**	.42***	.13	.29***
R Square	.64	.73	.75	.75	.55	.78	.74	.64	.71	.72	.74	.68	.69	.71
Number of questionnaires collected	**176**	**173**	**165**	**168**	**143**	**166**	**152**	**152**	**129**	**116**	**162**	**155**	**155**	**2012**

Note: ***p<.001; **p<.01; *p<.05.

To examine how the subject, class and teacher attributes subscales contributed to the global evaluation of the teacher (Item 11) and the course (Item 12), multiple regression analyses were carried out for the data collected from each lecture. Results of multiple regression analyses showed that the subject, class situation and teacher predicted global evaluation of the teacher and lecture (Table 4). For Item 11, teacher attributes was the strongest predictor. In contrast, subject attributes was the strongest predictor for Item 12. These findings provided support for the construct validity of the measure.

DISCUSSION

This study focused on the post-lecture subjective outcome evaluation of the subject entitled "Tomorrow's Leaders" offered at The Hong Kong Polytechnic University in the second piloting exercise. Similar to the first piloting exercise, the findings showed that the subject was very well received by the students. In particular, several observations can be highlighted from the findings. First, the subject, class and teacher attributes were perceived in a positive manner by the students. Second, compared with the first piloting exercise, the ratings in the second piloting exercise were higher. In conjunction with other evaluation strategies, the findings in these two piloting exercises clearly show that this subject was able to promote the holistic development of the students taking this subject.

Concerning the psychometric properties of the 10-item post-lecture subjective outcome evaluation form, factor analyses showed that three factors could be extracted from the scale, including subject, class and teacher attributes. This finding is in line with the original conceptual framework. Furthermore, reliability of the total scale and the related subscales were on the high side. As there is a severe lack of validated measures of evaluation tools in the Chinese culture (25), the present study is a positive response to the deficiency in the literature. Furthermore, with reference to the comment of Royse (26) that the use of validated measures of client satisfaction would "eliminate many of the problems found in hastily designed questionnaires" (p. 265), the present study is a contribution to the literature.

Finally, regarding predictors of perceived effectiveness of the course based on the data collected in different lectures, findings showed that subject, class and teacher attributes predicted global evaluation of the teacher, although their relative important differed for different dependent variables. For global evaluation of the teacher, the Teacher Attributes subscale was the strongest predictor. On the other hand, for global evaluation of the subject, The Subject Attributes subscale was the strongest predictor. This observation provides some support for the construct validity of the scale. With reference to the criticism of Durlak and DuPre (21) that the relative importance of different predictors of program effectiveness was inadequately examined, the present study is clearly a constructive response to this criticism.

Although the present study is pioneer in the field, it is noteworthy that there are some limitations of this study. First, only four classes of students were involved in this study. Hence, it would be helpful if more piloting exercises based on students in diverse populations could be conducted. Second, although the factors were consistent in Study 1 and Study 2, eigen value of the third factor was not high and a two-factor solution is not a suitable one. Hence, there is a need to further examine the factor structure of the post-lecture evaluation questionnaire in future. Third, although there are findings showing that the correlation between objective outcome evaluation and subjective outcome evaluation findings may be high (25), there is a need to examine this relationship in future studies.

ACKNOWLEDGMENTS

This work and the course on "Tomorrow's Leaders" are financially supported by The Hong Kong Polytechnic University. Members of the Curriculum Development Team included Daniel Shek, Yat Hung Chui, Siu Wai Lit, Yida Chung, Sowa Ngai, Yammy Chak, Pik Fong Tsui, Cecilia Ma, Lu Yu and Moon Law. This chapter has been published as a paper in the International Journal on Disability and Human Development, 2013;12(2). Permission has been obtained from De Gruyter to re-publish in this modified form.

REFERENCES

[1] Shek DTL. Nurturing holistic development of university students in Hong Kong: where are we and where should we go? Scientific World Journal 2010;10:563-75.

[2] Tsui YY, Wing YK. A study on the sleep patterns and problems of university business students in Hong Kong. J Am Coll Health 2009;58:167-76.

[3] Sing CY, Wong WS. Prevalence of insomnia and its psychosocial correlates among college students in Hong Kong. J Am Coll Health 2010;59:174-82.

[4] Kim JH, Chan WC, Chow JK, Fung KP, Fong BY, Cheuk KK, Griffiths S. University binge drinking patterns and changes in patterns of alcohol consumption among Chinese undergraduates in a Hong Kong university. J Am Coll Health 2009;58:255-65.

[5] Kim JH, Lau CH, Cheuk KK, Kan P, Hui HL, Griffiths SM. Brief report: predictors of heavy internet use and associations with health-promoting and health risk behaviors among Hong Kong university students. J Adolesc 2010;33:215-20.

[6] Tjosvold D, Nibler R, Wan P. Motivation for conflict among Chinese university students: effects of others' expertise and one's own confidence on engaging in conflict. J Soc Psychol 2001;141:353-63.

[7] Chan KL, Tiwari A, Leung WC, Ho HW, Cerulli C. Common correlates of suicidal ideation and physical assault among male and female university students in Hong Kong. Violence Vict 2007;22:290-303.

[8] Shek DTL, Wong KK. Do adolescent developmental issues disappear overnight? Reflections about holistic development in university students. ScientificWorldJournal 2011;11:353-61.

[9] Catalano RF, Berglund ML, Ryan JAM, Lonczak HS, Hawkins JD. Positive youth development in the United States: research findings on evaluations of positive youth development programs. Ann Am Pol Soc Sci 2004;591:98-124.

[10] Shek DTL, Yu L. Longitudinal impact of the Project P.A.T.H.S. on adolescent risk behavior: what happened after five years? ScientificWorldJournal 2012, Article ID 316029, 13 pages. DOI: 10.1100/2012/316029.

[11] Sun RCF, Shek DTL. Positive youth development, life satisfaction and problem behavior among Chinese adolescents in Hong Kong: a replication. Soc Indic Res 2012;105:541-59.

[12] Shek DTL. Qualitative evaluation of Project P.A.T.H.S. in Hong Kong: focus groups based on Secondary 3 program implementers. Int J Adolesc Med Health 2012;24:245-52.

[13] Shek DTL, Ma CMS, Kan VWM. Subjective outcome evaluation of Project P.A.T.H.S. based on different cohorts of students. Int J Disabil Hum Dev 2011;10:227-34.

[14] Shek DTL, Ma CMS, Tang CYP. Predictors of subjective outcome evaluation findings in a positive youth development program in Hong Kong. Int J Disabil Hum Dev 2011;10:249-55.

[15] Shek DTL, Sun RCF, Merrick J. Editorial: how to promote holistic development in university students? Int J Disabil Hum Dev 2012;11:171-2.
[16] Shek DTL. Development of a positive youth development subject in a university context in Hong Kong. Int J Disabil Hum Dev 2012;11:173-9.
[17] Shek DTL, Sun RCF. Promoting psychosocial competencies in university students: evaluation based on a one group pretest-posttest design. Int J Disabil Hum Dev 2012;11:229-34.
[18] Shek DTL, Sun RCF. Promoting leadership and intrapersonal competence in university students: what can we learn from Hong Kong? Int J Disabil Hum Dev 2012;11:221-8.
[19] Shek DTL, Sun RCF. Process evaluation of a positive youth development course in a university setting in Hong Kong. Int J Disabil Hum Dev 2012;11:235-41.
[20] Shek DTL, Sun RCF. Qualitative evaluation of a positive youth development course in a university setting in Hong Kong. Int J Disabil Hum Dev 2012:11:243-8.
[21] Shek DTL, Sun RCF. Focus group evaluation of a positive youth development course in a university in Hong Kong. Int J Disabil Hum Dev 2012;11:249-54.
[22] Shek DTL, Sun RCF, Chui YH, Lit SW, Yuen WW, Chung Y, Ngai SW. Development and evaluation of a positive youth development course for university students in Hong Kong. ScientificWorldJournal 2012, Article ID 263731, 8 pages. DOI: 10.1100/2012/263731.
[23] Shek DTL. Post-lecture evaluation of a positive youth development subject for university students in Hong Kong. ScientificWorldJournal 2012, Article ID 934679, 8 pages. DOI: 10.1100/2012/934679.
[24] Shek DTL, Wu FKY. Reflective journals of students taking a positive youth development course in a university context in Hong Kong. ScientificWorldJournal 2012, Article ID 131560, 8 pages. DOI: 10.1100/2012/131560.
[25] Shek DTL. Subjective outcome and objective outcome evaluation findings: insights from a Chinese context. Res Soc Work Pract 2010;20:293-301.
[26] Royse D. Research methods in social work. Pacific Grove, CA: Brooks/Cole-Thomson Learning, 2004.
[27] Durlak JA, DuPre EP. Implementation matters: a review of research on the influence of implementation on program outcomes and the factors affecting implementation. Am J Commun Psychol 2008;41:327-50.

In: Chinese Adolescent Development ISBN: 978-1-62618-622-4
Editors: Daniel TL Shek, Rachel CF Sun, Joav Merrick © 2013 Nova Science Publishers, Inc.

Chapter 9

POST-COURSE SUBJECTIVE OUTCOME EVALUATION OF A COURSE PROMOTING LEADERSHIP AND INTRAPERSONAL DEVELOPMENT IN UNIVERSITY STUDENTS IN HONG KONG

***Daniel TL Shek*[*,1,2,3,4,5]**
***and Rachel CF Sun*[6]**

[1]Department of Applied Social Sciences,
The Hong Kong Polytechnic University, Hong Kong, PRC
[2]Centre for Innovative Programmes for Adolescents and Families The Hong Kong Polytechnic University, Hong Kong, PRC
[3]Kiang Wu Nursing College of Macau, Macau, PRC
[4]Department of Social Work, East China Normal University, Shanghai, PRC
[5]Division of Adolescent Medicine, Department of Pediatrics,
Kentucky Children's Hospital, University of Kentucky College of Medicine, Lexington, Kentucky, US
[6]Faculty of Education, The University of Hong Kong, Hong Kong, PRC

ABSTRACT

Two studies were conducted to examine the psychometric properties of the 37-item Subjective Outcome Evaluation Scale (SOES) developed to evaluate the subject, instructor and benefits of a course on leadership and intrapersonal development at The Hong Kong Polytechnic University. Consistent with the conceptual framework, factor analyses in both studies (N = 268 and N = 195, respectively) showed that three factors (course, instructor and benefits) were abstracted from the scale. In Study 2, the SOES was found to be internally consistent and the different sub-scales were significantly correlated amongst themselves. Both perceived qualities of the program and instructor

* Correspondence: Professor Daniel TL Shek, PhD, FHKPS, BBS, JP, Chair Professor of Applied Social Sciences, Faculty of Health and Social Sciences, Department of Applied Social Sciences, The Hong Kong Polytechnic University, Room HJ407, Core H, Hunghom, Hong Kong. E-mail: daniel.shek@polyu.edu.hk

were significant predictors of the perceived effectiveness of the program. Consistent with Study 1, results in Study 2 showed that the students generally had positive perceptions of the program and implementers, with over 90% of the participants indicating that they were satisfied with the program.

INTRODUCTION

In the field of human service, accountability is an important issue to be considered. Hence, evaluation is strongly emphasized in different professions such as social work and education, particularly with reference to evidence-based approach. While it is desirable to conduct clinical trials to study the effectiveness of programs, it is not always possible to do this because of the complexity and huge resources involved in such an evaluation strategy. From the practitioners' point of view, it is necessary to have a handy and convenient way to assess program effectiveness. For instance, the client satisfaction approach or subjective outcome evaluation is commonly used by human professionals to evaluate social programs. The common mode is to use a client satisfaction scale with both closed-ended and open-ended questions to assess the subjective perceptions of the program participants, instructors and benefits of the program. For example, subjective outcome evaluation has been used in a large scale positive youth development program entitled Project P.A.T.H.S. in Hong Kong (1-5). The common mode of evaluation is that the students are required to complete a subjective outcome evaluation form on three dimensions (program, instructor and benefits) after attending the course.

Methodologically speaking, subjective outcome evaluation enjoys the ease of administration, the ease of data analysis, economic efficiency and capability of capturing the program participants' perspective. Nevertheless, subjective outcome evaluation has been criticized as unscientific because the related data are usually skewed toward the positive pole. Furthermore, the correlation between subjective outcome evaluation and objective outcome evaluation may not be high (6). As pointed out by Royse (7), "despite the generally positive bias and the problems associated with collecting representative samples of clients, there is much to recommend client satisfaction studies as one means of evaluating a program. Because professionals do not experience the agency in the same way as the clients, it is important to ask clients to share their experiences" (p. 264-265). Although there are many factors contributing to the possible biases in subjective outcome evaluation, the lack of standardized subjective outcome evaluation measures is an important factor to be considered. Hence, it is important to develop assessment tools with sound psychometric properties.

With particular reference to the Chinese culture, although subjective outcome evaluation is commonly used in human services, sound instruments are not pervasive in the welfare settings. Nevertheless, some validated measures of student feedback questionnaires in the higher education sector do exist. For example, Kember and Leung (8) identified nine dimensions in the Exemplary Teacher Course Questionnaire (ETCQ), including understanding fundamental concepts, relevance, challenging beliefs, active learning, teacher-student relationships, motivation, organization, flexibility, and assessment. There is also support for the dimensions of the Chinese version of the Students' Evaluations of Educational Quality developed by Marsh and Roche (9), including learning/value, teacher enthusiasm, organization/clarity, group interaction, individual rapport, breadth of coverage, examinations/grading, assignments/readings, and workload/difficulty (10, 11). Unfortunately, perceived benefits of the course are usually not asked in depth in these assessment tools.

The purpose of this chapter is to report findings on the psychometric properties of the Subjective Outcome Evaluation Scale (SOES) in a university context. Under the new Undergraduate Curriculum, The Hong Kong Polytechnic University will require all students to take a course on Leadership and Intrapersonal Development starting from the 2012/13 academic year. A subject entitled "Tomorrow's Leaders" has been developed to fulfill this requirement. In this course, different positive youth developmental constructs, including self-understanding, resilience, cognitive competence, social competence, emotional competence, moral competence, integrity, spirituality, clear and positive identity, will be promoted to university students. To test out the curriculum, "Tomorrow's Leaders" was offered in the second term of the 2010/11 academic year on a pilot basis. While the evaluation findings based on the Subjective Outcome Evaluation Scale were very encouraging, dimensionality of the scale was not reported in the associated paper (12). As the subject was piloted again in the first term of the 2011/12 academic year, it is a good opportunity to examine the psychometric properties of the scale. Besides, degree of satisfaction of the students and predictors of perceived effectiveness were examined in this study.

STUDY 1

Methods

In the second term of the 2010/11 academic year, the subject "Tomorrow's Leaders" was offered to 268 students in four classes (N = 268). At the last lecture of the course, students were invited to respond to a subjective outcome evaluation form. On the day of data collection, the purpose of the evaluation was mentioned, and confidentiality of the data was repeatedly emphasized to all students. The students were asked to indicate their wish if they did not want to participate in the study (i.e., "passive" informed consent was obtained from the students). All participants responded to all scales in the evaluation form in a self-administration format. Adequate time was provided for the participants to complete the questionnaire.

Instruments

The subjective outcome form used in this study was modeled after the Subjective Outcome Evaluation Form for students (Form A) of the Project P.A.T.H.S. in Hong Kong. Broadly speaking, there are several parts in this evaluation form as follows:

- Participants' perceptions of the program, such as program objectives, design, classroom atmosphere, interaction among the students, and the respondents' participation during class (10 items).
- Participants' perceptions of the implementers, such as the preparation of the lecturer, professional attitude, involvement, and interaction with the students (10 items).

- Participants' perceptions of the effectiveness of the program (such as promotion of different psychosocial competencies, resilience, and overall personal development) and achievement of the intended learning outcomes (17 items).
- The extent to which the participants would recommend the program to other people with similar needs (1 item).
- The extent to which the participants would join similar programs in the future (1 item).
- Overall satisfaction with the program (1 item).
- Things that the participants learned from the program (open-ended question).
- Things that the participants appreciated most (open-ended question).
- Opinion about the instructor(s) (open-ended question).
- Areas that require improvement (open-ended question).

With reference to the subject, instructor and effectiveness in the conceptual model, it was hypothesized that three factors would be extracted from the related 37 items, including perceptions of the subject, teacher and effectiveness.

Results and discussion

A total of 189 subjective outcome evaluation forms were collected at the last lecture of the course. To provide an empirical summary of the data collected and to extract the maximum amount of variance from the data set with some orthogonal components, a principal components analysis was carried out for each factor analysis followed by varimax rotation. A principal components analysis was performed on the participants' responses to the SOES, yielding four factors with eigenvalues exceeding unity, explaining 65.5% of the variance.

To avoid over-factoring, further analyses using the scree test showed that three factors could be meaningfully extracted. The three-factor solution, which could be considered as relatively adequate representations of the data, was rotated to a varimax criterion for interpretation.

The first factor, which could be labeled Benefits, included Items 21 to 37. These items are basically concerned with perceptions of the benefits and this factor explained 30.89% of the variance. The second factor, which included Items 11 to 20 could be labeled Teacher factor, accounting for 18.65% of the variance. Factor III explained 15.95% of the total variance, which included Items 1 to 10. Because these items are concerned with perceptions of the subject and its implementation, this factor could hence be labeled a Subject factor. The varimax rotated factor structure based on the total sample can be seen in Table 1.

Consistent with the hypothesized conceptual model, three dimensions were abstracted from the scale. As reported by Shek and Sun (12), the related subscales were internally consistent. However, because of the small sample involved, it is not possible to assess the stability of the factor structure. Therefore, it is desirable to replicate the findings in another sample and examine the stability of the factor structure across different samples.

Table 1. Factor structure of the Chinese Subjective Outcome Evaluation Scale in Study 1

Item		Factor 1	Factor 2	Factor 3
1	Objectives of the curriculum are very clear.	.402	.279	**.589**
2	Design of the curriculum is very good.	.434	.335	**.666**
3	Activities were carefully arranged.	.342	.372	**.647**
4	Classroom atmosphere was very pleasant.	.373	.187	**.700**
5	Peer interaction amongst the students.	.281	.126	**.748**
6	I participated actively during lessons.	.217	.177	**.807**
7	I was encouraged to do my best.	.348	.209	**.643**
8	Enhanced my interest towards the lessons.	.493	.247	**.613**
9	I have very positive evaluation of the program.	.477	.284	**.588**
10	I like this curriculum very much.	.566	.206	**.605**
11	The lecturer(s) had a good mastery of the curriculum.	.186	**.734**	.123
12	The lecturer(s) was (were) well prepared for the lessons.	.183	**.768**	.037
13	The teaching skills of the lecturer(s) were good.	.396	**.637**	.204
14	The lecturer(s) showed good professional attitudes.	.134	**.851**	.162
15	The lecturer(s) was (were) very involved.	.080	**.792**	.210
16	The lecturer(s) encouraged students to participate.	-.001	**.778**	.224
17	The lecturer(s) cared for the students.	.197	**.771**	.138
18	The lecturer(s) was (were) ready to offer help.	.168	**.715**	.145
19	The lecturer(s) had much interaction with the students.	.213	**.676**	.222
20	I have very positive evaluation of the lecturer(s).	.128	**.854**	.175
21	Strengthened my resilience in adverse conditions.	**.833**	.166	.202
22	Enhanced my social competence.	**.724**	.212	.264
23	Improved my ability in expressing and handling my emotions.	**.807**	.102	.225
24	Enhanced my analytical ability.	**.758**	.139	.280
25	Improved my ability to resist harmful influences.	**.751**	.168	.216
26	Strengthened my ability to distinguish between the good and the bad.	**.810**	.195	.193
27	Increased my competence in making sensible and wise choices.	**.822**	.139	.163
28	Helped me to have life reflections.	**.700**	.232	.290
29	Strengthened my self-confidence.	**.804**	.098	.303
30	Increased my self-awareness.	**.719**	.127	.368
31	Helped me to face the future with a positive attitude.	**.799**	.123	.327
32	Helped me to cultivate compassion and care about others.	**.798**	.094	.163
33	Enabled me to understand successful leaders.	**.568**	.209	.168
34	Helped me synthesize the characteristics of successful leaders.	**.653**	.259	.230

Table 1. (Continued)

Item		Factor 1	Factor 2	Factor 3
35	Enabled me to understand the importance of interpersonal relationship.	**.567**	.127	.312
36	Promoted my sense of responsibility in serving the society.	**.681**	.170	.324
37	Enriched my overall development.	**.778**	.186	.339
Eigen Value		13.98	4.39	1.87
Variance Explained		30.89	18.65	15.95

The highest loading amongst the factors for an item is marked in bold. Factor 1 = Perceived effectiveness of the program; Factor 2 = Perceived instructor qualities; Factor 3 = Perceived program qualities.

STUDY 2

Methods

In the first term of the 2011/12 academic year, the subject “Tomorrow’s Leaders” was offered to 195 students in four classes. At the last lecture of the course, students were invited to respond to a subjective outcome evaluation form. The Subject Outcome Evaluation Scale (SOES) used in Study 1 was adopted in this study.

Results

A total of 142 subjective outcome evaluation forms were collected at the last lecture of the course. A principal components analysis was performed on the participants' responses to the SOES, yielding four factors with eigenvalues exceeding unity, explaining 62.59% of the variance. To avoid over-factoring, further analyses using the scree test showed that three factors could be meaningfully extracted. The three-factor solution, which could be considered as relatively adequate representations of the data, was rotated to a varimax criterion for interpretation. These included the Benefits factor (Items 21 to 37; 25.17%), Subject factor (Item 1 to Item 10; 22.19%) and Teacher factors (Item 11 to Item 20; 15.23%). The varimax rotated factor structure based on the total sample can be seen in Table 2. To examine the stability of the factor structure of the SOES across studies, coefficients of congruence amongst the corresponding factors in Study 1 and Study 2 were computed: Benefits = 0.98, Teacher = 0.90, Subject = 0.92. These findings demonstrated that the dimensionality of the factors was consistent across studies.

Reliability analysis showed that the subjective outcome evaluation form was internally consistent (Table 3): 10 items related to the program (α = .94), 10 items related to the implementer (α = .93), 17 items related to the benefits (α = .95), and the overall 37 items measuring program effectiveness (α = .97). As such, a composite measure of each domain (i.e., perceived qualities of program content, perceived qualities of program implementers, and perceived program effectiveness) was created based on the total scores of each factor divided by the number of items in that domain. Pearson correlation analysis was used to examine if the three dimensions were inter correlated. Multiple regression analysis was performed to compare which factor would predict the program effectiveness.

Table 2. Factor structure of the Chinese Subjective Outcome Evaluation Scale in Study 2

Item		Factor 1	Factor 2	Factor 3
1	Objectives of the curriculum are very clear.	.256	**.690**	.290
2	Design of the curriculum is very good.	.346	**.772**	.217
3	Activities were carefully arranged.	.277	**.765**	.302
4	Classroom atmosphere was very pleasant.	.215	**.750**	.233
5	Peer interaction amongst the students.	.196	**.672**	.327
6	I participated actively during lessons.	.245	**.634**	.206
7	I was encouraged to do my best.	.423	**.625**	.246
8	Enhanced my interest towards the lessons.	.528	**.600**	.195
9	I have very positive evaluation of the program.	.305	**.737**	.252
10	I like this curriculum very much.	.386	**.745**	.144
11	The lecturer(s) had a good mastery of the curriculum.	.150	.381	**.679**
12	The lecturer(s) was (were) well prepared for the lessons.	.028	.410	**.671**
13	The teaching skills of the lecturer(s) were good.	.225	.546	**.539**
14	The lecturer(s) showed good professional attitudes.	.099	.318	**.726**
15	The lecturer(s) was (were) very involved.	.190	.379	**.705**
16	The lecturer(s) encouraged students to participate.	.156	.467	**.535**
17	The lecturer(s) cared for the students.	.281	.590	**.437**
18	The lecturer(s) was (were) ready to offer help.	.251	.479	**.519**
19	The lecturer(s) had much interaction with the students.	.310	.579	**.445**
20	I have very positive evaluation of the lecturer(s).	.276	.615	**.492**
21	Strengthened my resilience in adverse conditions.	**.704**	.274	-.024
22	Enhanced my social competence.	**.625**	.295	.097
23	Improved my ability in expressing and handling my emotions.	**.804**	.195	.155
24	Enhanced my analytical ability.	**.667**	.235	.154
25	Improved my ability to resist harmful influences.	**.763**	.189	.055
26	Strengthened my ability to distinguish between the good and the bad.	**.766**	.224	.169
27	Increased my competence in making sensible and wise choices.	**.760**	.254	.035
28	Helped me to have life reflections.	**.630**	.321	.210
29	Strengthened my self-confidence.	**.765**	.199	.239
30	Increased my self-awareness.	**.616**	.218	.365
31	Helped me to face the future with a positive attitude.	**.643**	.158	.374
32	Helped me to cultivate compassion and care about others.	**.659**	.227	.303
33	Enabled me to understand successful leaders.	**.512**	.107	.588

Table 2. (Continued)

Item		Factor 1	Factor 2	Factor 3
34	Helped me synthesize the characteristics of successful leaders.	**.565**	.117	.585
35	Enabled me to understand the importance of interpersonal relationship.	**.546**	.152	.548
36	Promoted my sense of responsibility in serving the society.	**.684**	.344	.179
37	Enriched my overall development.	**.686**	.290	.189
Eigen Value		18.18	3.34	1.63
Variance Explained		25.17	22.19	15.23

The highest loading amongst the factors for an item is marked in bold. Factor 1 = Perceived effectiveness of the program; Factor 2 = Perceived instructor qualities; Factor 3 = Perceived program qualities.

Results of correlation analyses showed that both program content ($r = .71$, $p < .01$) and program implementers ($r = .64$, $p < .01$) were strongly associated with program effectiveness (Table 4). Table 5 presents multiple regression analysis results. Findings showed that both program content and program implementer were found to be significant predictors of perceived program effectiveness when other factors were controlled.

Table 3. Mean, standard deviations, Cronbach's alphas, and mean of inter-item correlations among the variables

	Overall	
	M (SD)	**α (Mean[#])**
Program content (10 items)	5.11 (.58)	.94 (.63)
Program implementers (10 items)	5.26 (.50)	.93 (.58)
Program effectiveness (17 items)	4.08 (.56)	.95 (.54)
Total effectiveness (37 items)	4.68 (.48)	.97 (.48)

[#] Mean inter-item correlations.

Table 4. Correlation coefficients among the variables

Variable	**1**	**2**	**3**	**4**
1. Program content (10 items)	-			
2. Program implementers (10 items)	.81**	-		
3. Program effectiveness (17 items)	.71**	.64**	-	
4. Total effectiveness (37 items)	.91**	.87**	.91**	-

$^{**}p < .01$.

Table 5. Multiple regression analyses predicting program effectiveness

	Predictors		Model	
	Program content	Program implementers		
	ß[a]	ß[a]	R	R^2
Program effectiveness	.53**	.21*	.72	.51

[a] Standardized coefficients.
*$p < .05$, **$p < .01$.

The quantitative findings based on the closed-ended questions are presented in this chapter. Several observations can be highlighted from the findings. In the first place, over 95% of the participants had positive perceptions of the course (Table 6), including clear objectives of the curriculum (99.3%), well-planned teaching activities (98.59%), and adequate peer interaction among the students (98.59%). In addition, a high proportion of the students had positive evaluation of the implementers (Table 7). For example, all participants perceived that the implementers had well preparation for the lessons, were very involved, and encouraged students to participate in the activities. Regarding the perceived effectiveness of the course (Table 8), 100% of students believed that the course had helped them to understand the qualities of effective leadership as well as enabled them to understand the importance of interpersonal relationship in successful leadership. Over 97% of the respondents perceived that the program promoted their development. Finally, more than 99% of the participants indicated that they were satisfied with the course (Table 9).

DISCUSSION

One of the objectives of this study was to examine the dimensionality of the Subjective Outcome Evaluation Scale (SOES). Consistent with the conceptual framework, three aspects of the scale, including subject, teacher and effectiveness were identified through factor analyses and the factors were consistent across samples. Besides, reliability analyses showed that the total scale and the subscales were found to be internally consistent. Furthermore, the significant inter-correlation amongst the subscales also provided some support for the construct validity of the SOES. In view of the lack of subjective outcome evaluation measures in the Chinese human service context, the present study is an interesting contribution to the Chinese literature on subjective outcome evaluation. According to Royse (7), client satisfaction surveys are commonly criticized as invalid because there is a lack of standardized assessment tools for conducting subjective outcome evaluation. As such, he suggested using subjective outcome evaluation tools with good psychometric properties which would "eliminate many of the problems found in hastily designed questionnaires" (p. 265). Therefore, the present study is a constructive response to the limitation of the literature.

Regarding the prediction of perceived effectiveness of the subject, findings showed that both subject and teacher were significant predictors. There are two interesting observations that can be highlighted from the findings. First, the finding that both subject and teacher were significant predictors of perceived effectiveness is inconsistent with the previous finding that teacher was not a significant predictor of perceived effectiveness of the subject (12).

Table 6. Summary of the views of the program participants of the program (N=142)

	1 Strongly Disagree		2 Disagree		3 Slightly Disagree		4 Slightly Agree		5 Agree		6 Strongly Agree		Participants with Positive Response (options 4-6)	
	N	%	N	%	N	%	N	%	N	%	N	%	N	%
1. The objectives of the curriculum are very clear.	0	0	0	0	1	0.70	18	12.68	87	61.27	36	25.35	141	99.30
2. The design of the curriculum is very good.	0	0	1	0.70	3	2.11	21	14.79	81	57.04	36	25.35	138	97.18
3. The activities were carefully arranged.	0	0	0	0	2	1.41	22	15.49	77	54.23	41	28.87	140	98.59
4. The classroom atmosphere was very pleasant.	0	0	0	0	4	2.82	14	9.86	77	54.23	47	33.10	138	97.18
5. There was much peer interaction amongst the students.	0	0	0	0	2	1.41	13	9.15	73	51.41	54	38.03	140	98.59
6. I participated actively during lessons (including discussions, sharing, games, etc.).	0	0	0	0	3	2.11	21	14.79	79	55.63	39	27.46	139	97.89
7. I was encouraged to do my best.	0	0	0	0	3	2.11	26	18.31	80	56.34	33	23.24	139	97.89
8. The learning experience I encountered enhanced my interest towards the lessons.	0	0	0	0	5	3.52	24	16.90	75	52.82	38	26.76	137	96.48
9. Overall speaking, I have very positive evaluation of the program.	0	0	0	0	2	1.41	25	17.61	71	50.00	44	30.99	140	98.59
10. On the whole, I like this curriculum very much.	0	0	1	0.70	1	0.70	16	11.27	76	53.52	48	33.80	140	98.59

Table 7. Summary of the views of the teachers implementing the program (N=142)

	1 Strongly Disagree		2 Disagree		3 Slightly Disagree		4 Slightly Agree		5 Agree		6 Strongly Agree		Participants with Positive Response (options 4-6)	
	N	%	N	%	N	%	N	%	N	%	N	%	N	%
1. The lecturer(s) had a good mastery of the curriculum.	0	0	0	0	2	1.41	9	6.34	89	62.68	42	29.58	140	98.59
2. The lecturer (s) was well prepared for the lessons.	0	0	0	0	0	0	9	6.34	78	54.93	55	38.73	142	100
3. The teaching skills of the lecturer were good.	0	0	0	0	1	0.70	20	14.08	73	51.41	48	33.80	141	99.30
4. The lecturer (s) showed good professional attitudes.	0	0	0	0	1	0.70	5	3.52	86	60.56	50	35.21	141	99.30
5. The lecturer(s) was very involved.	0	0	0	0	0	0	8	5.63	77	54.23	57	40.14	142	100
6. The lecturer (s) encouraged students to participate in the activities.	0	0	0	0	0	0	15	10.56	66	46.48	61	42.96	142	100
7. The instructor cared for the students.	0	0	1	0.70	0	0	17	11.97	74	52.11	50	35.21	141	99.30
8. The lecturer(s) was ready to offer help to students when needed.	0	0	0	0	1	0.70	13	9.15	79	55.63	49	34.51	141	99.30
9. The lecturer(s) had much interaction with the students.	0	0	0	0	1	0.70	19	13.38	73	51.41	49	34.51	141	99.30
10. Overall speaking, I have very positive evaluation of the lecturer(s).	0	0	0	0	0	0	13	9.15	77	54.23	52	36.62	142	100

Table 8. Perceived effectiveness of the program by the program participants (N=142)

The extent to which the course (i.e., the program that all students have joined) has helped you:	1 Unhelpful		2 Not Very Helpful		3 Slightly Helpful		4 Helpful		5 Very Helpful		Participants with Positive Response (options 3-5)	
	N	%	N	%	N	%	N	%	N	%	N	%
1. It has strengthened my resilience in adverse conditions.	0	0	3	2.11	23	16.20	85	59.86	31	21.83	139	97.89
2. It has enhanced my social competence.	0	0	1	0.70	15	10.56	88	61.97	38	26.76	141	99.30
3. It has improved my ability in handling and expressing my emotions.	0	0	1	0.70	21	14.79	86	60.56	34	23.94	141	99.30
4. It has enhanced my analytical ability.	0	0	3	2.11	32	22.54	78	54.93	29	20.42	139	97.89
5. It has improved my ability to resist harmful influences.	0	0	3	2.11	30	21.13	78	54.93	31	21.83	139	97.89
6. It has strengthened my ability to distinguish between the good and the bad.	0	0	3	2.11	28	19.72	72	50.70	39	27.46	139	97.89
7. It has increased my competence in making sensible and wise choices.	0	0	2	1.41	28	19.72	80	56.34	32	22.54	140	98.59
8. It has helped me to have life reflections.	0	0	1	0.70	15	10.56	72	50.70	54	38.03	141	99.30
9. It has reinforced my self-confidence.	0	0	5	3.52	24	16.90	84	59.15	29	20.42	137	96.48
10. It has increased my self-awareness.	0	0	1	0.70	16	11.27	75	52.82	50	35.21	141	99.30
11. It has helped me to face the future with a positive attitude.	0	0	1	0.70	23	16.20	77	54.23	41	28.87	141	99.30
12. It has helped me to cultivate compassion and care about others.	0	0	4	2.82	30	21.13	77	54.23	31	21.83	138	97.18
13. The theories, research and concepts covered in the course have enabled me to understand the characteristics of successful leaders.	0	0	0	0	15	10.64	84	59.57	42	29.79	141	100
14. The course has helped me synthesize the characteristics of successful leaders.	0	0	1	0.70	22	15.49	80	56.34	39	27.46	141	99.30
15. It has enabled me to understand the importance of interpersonal relationship in successful leadership.	0	0	0	0	16	11.27	85	59.86	41	28.87	142	100
16. It has promoted my sense of responsibility in serving the society.	0	0	6	4.23	28	19.72	71	50.00	37	26.06	136	95.77
17. It has enriched my overall development.	0	0	3	2.11	19	13.38	74	52.11	46	32.39	139	97.88

Table 9. Other aspects of subjective outcome evaluation

Will you suggest your friends to take this course? (N=142)

1 Definitely Will Not Suggest		2 Will Not Suggest		3 Will Suggest		4 Definitely Will Suggest		Participants with Positive Response (options 3-4)	
N	%	N	%	N	%	N	%	N	%
0	0	5	3.52	91	64.08	46	32.39	137	96.48

Will you participate in similar courses again in the future? (N=142)

1 Definitely Will Not Participate		2 Will Not Participate		3 Will Participate		4 Definitely Will Participate		Participants with Positive Response (options 3-4)	
N	%	N	%	N	%	N	%	N	%
1	0.70	21	14.79	86	60.56	34	23.94	120	84.51

On the whole, are you satisfied with this course? (N=141)

1 Very Dissatisfied		2 Moderately Dissatisfied		3 Slightly Dissatisfied		4 Satisfied		5 Moderately Satisfied		6 Very Satisfied		Participants with Positive Response (options 4-6)	
N	%	N	%	N	%	N	%	N	%	N	%	N	%
0	0	0	0	1	0.71	37	26.24	69	48.94	34	24.11	140	99.29

On the other hand, the present study is in line with the finding that both program and teacher were significant predictors of program effectiveness (13). This observation supports the idea that effectiveness of implementation is multidimensional (14). Second, contrary to common sense beliefs, program was found to be more powerful in predicting perceived effectiveness. There are two possible explanations for this observation. First, as the distribution of scores for the teacher factor was not wide, the ceiling effect may contribute to its weaker impact on perceived effectiveness (i.e., the finding is due to statistical artifact).

Second, it is possible that the students are differentiating in their views of the program features and effectiveness so that they would not blindly give good scores on effectiveness even if the teachers were not good.

Consistent with the findings in Study 1, the subjective outcome evaluation findings showed that the participants had very positive perceptions of the subject and teachers. In particular, the finding showed that the perceived benefits of the subject were very great. The findings are in line with the findings in Shek and Sun (12) and the positive effects were even higher than the first piloting exercise. In conjunction with other evaluation findings, the findings strongly suggest that "Tomorrow's Leaders" is a subject which can promote the leadership and intrapersonal development of students. With reference to the growing concerns about developmental issues in university students (15-20), the available research findings suggest that the developed course is a promising response.

It is noteworthy that there are several possible explanations of the positive evaluation findings. The first explanation is that the program was effective in promoting the holistic development of university students. Second, it can be argued that the students responded positively because they were afraid of being punished by the teachers concerned. However, this alternative explanation is not plausible because the students responded in an anonymous manner. Finally, "demand characteristic" of the respondents (i.e., they attempted to please the teachers) may explain the overall positive findings. However, this alternative explanation can also be partially dismissed because students were encouraged to respond in an honest manner and there is no reason why the students should please the teachers.

ACKNOWLEDGMENTS

This work and the course on "Tomorrow's Leaders" are financially supported by The Hong Kong Polytechnic University. Members of the Curriculum Development Team include Daniel T.L. Shek, Y.H. Chui, S.W. Lit, Yida Y.H. Chung, Sowa S.W. Ngai, Yammy L.Y. Chak, P.F. Tsui, Cecilia M.S. Ma, Lu Yu and Moon Y.M. Law. This chapter has been published as a paper in the International Journal on Disability and Human Development, 2013;12(2). Permission has been obtained from De Gruyter to re-publish in this modified form.

REFERENCES

[1] Shek DTL, Ma CMS, Tang CYP. Predictors of subjective outcome evaluation findings in a positive youth development program in Hong Kong. Int J Disabil Hum Dev 2011;10:249-55.

[2] Shek DTL, Sun RCF, Merrick J. Training programs and implementation process of positive youth development programs. Int J Adolesc Med Health 2011;23:303-304.

[3] Shek DTL, Ma HK, Sun RCF. A brief overview of adolescent developmental problems in Hong Kong. ScientificWorldJournal 2011;11:2243-56.

[4] Shek DTL, Ma HK, Sun RCF. Development of a new curriculum in a positive youth development program: the Project P.A.T.H.S. in Hong Kong. ScientificWorldJournal 2011;11:2207-18.

[5] Shek DTL. Quality of life research: responses to emerging issues in a changing world. Soc Indic Res 2011;100:371-74.

[6] Shek DTL. Subjective outcome and objective outcome evaluation findings: insights from a Chinese context. Res Social Work Prac 2010;20:293-301.

[7] Royse D. Research methods in social work. Pacific Grove, CA: Brooks/Cole-Thomson Learning, 2004.

[8] Kember D, Leung DY. Establishing the validity and reliability of course evaluation questionnaires. Assessment and Evaluation in Higher Education 2008;33(4):341-53.

[9] Marsh HW, Roche LA. Making students' evaluations of teaching effectiveness effective: the critical issues of validity, bias and utility. Am Psychol 1997;52:1187-97.

[10] Marsh HW, Hau KT, Chung CM, Siu TL. Students' evaluations of university teaching: Chinese version of the students' evaluations of educational quality (SEEQ) instrument. J Educ Psychol 1997;89:568-72.

[11] Marsh HW, Hau KT, Chung CM, Siu TL. Confirmatory factor analysis of students' evaluations: Chinese SEEQ version. Structural Equation Modeling 1998;5:143-64.

[12] Shek DTL, Sun RCF. Promoting leadership and intrapersonal competence in university students: what can we learn from Hong Kong? Int J Disabil Hum Dev 2012;11:221-28.

[13] Shek DTL, Ma CMS. Subjective outcome evaluation findings: factors related to the perceived effectiveness of the Tier 2 Program of the Project P.A.T.H.S. ScientificWorldJournal 2010;10:250-60.

[14] Durlak JA, DuPre EP. Implementation matters: a review of research on the influence of implementation on program outcomes and the factors affecting implementation. Am J Commun Psychol 2008;41:327-50.
[15] Twenge JM, Konrath S, Foster JD, Campbell WK, Bushman BJ. Egos inflating over time: a cross-temporal metal-analysis of the narcissistic personality inventory. J Pers 2008;76:875-901.
[16] Twenge JM, Foster JD. Birth cohort increases in narcissistic personality traits among American college students, 1982–2009. Soc Psychol Personal Sci 2010;1:99-106.
[17] Bourke B, Mechler HS. A new me generation? The increasing self-interest among Millennial college students. J Coll Char 2010;11:1-6.
[18] Loeb PR. Generation at the crossroads: apathy and action on the American campus. New Brunswick, NJ: Rutgers University Press, 1994.
[19] Shek DTL. Nurturing holistic development of university students in Hong Kong: where are we and where should we go? ScientificWorldJournal 2010;10:563-75.
[20] Shek DTL, Wong KK. Do adolescent developmental issues disappear overnight? Reflections about holistic development in university students. ScientificWorldJournal 2011;11:353-61.

In: Chinese Adolescent Development ISBN: 978-1-62618-622-4
Editors: Daniel TL Shek, Rachel CF Sun, Joav Merrick © 2013 Nova Science Publishers, Inc.

Chapter 10

PROCESS EVALUATION OF A LEADERSHIP AND INTRAPERSONAL DEVELOPMENT SUBJECT FOR UNIVERSITY STUDENTS

***Daniel TL Shek**[*,1,2,3,4,5]* ***and Rachel CF Sun**[6]*

[1]Department of Applied Social Sciences,
The Hong Kong Polytechnic University, Hong Kong, PRC
[2]Centre for Innovative Programmes for Adolescents and Families,
The Hong Kong Polytechnic University, Hong Kong, PRC
[3]Kiang Wu Nursing College of Macau, Macau, PRC
[4]Department of Social Work, East China Normal University, Shanghai, PRC
[5]Division of Adolescent Medicine, Department of Pediatrics,
Kentucky Children's Hospital, University of Kentucky College of Medicine,
Lexington, Kentucky, US
[6]Faculty of Education, The University of Hong Kong,
Hong Kong, PRC

ABSTRACT

Under the New Undergraduate Curriculum, a subject entitled "Tomorrow's Leaders" was developed to enable students to fulfill the requirement in the area of Leadership and Intrapersonal Development at The Hong Kong Polytechnic University. In the second piloting exercise, process evaluation was carried out for 19 lectures, with each lecture observed by two independent observers. Results showed that inter-rater reliability was generally high. Regarding program implementation, findings showed that program adherence and implementation quality of the subject were high. It was also found that classroom management, time management and achievement of teaching unit's objectives were significant predictors of overall quality and success of the program. The present

[*] Correspondence: Professor Daniel TL Shek, PhD, FHKPS, BBS, JP, Chair Professor of Applied Social Sciences, Faculty of Health and Social Sciences, Department of Applied Social Sciences, The Hong Kong Polytechnic University, Room HJ407, Core H, Hunghom, Hong Kong. E-mail: daniel.shek@polyu.edu.hk

study reinforced the conclusion that the implementation quality of "Tomorrow's Leaders" was high.

INTRODUCTION

In view of the growing adolescent developmental problems in the global context, there is a call for the development of adolescent prevention and positive youth development programs. Nevertheless, a survey of the literature shows that such programs are not always successful. For example, Catalano et al. (1) found that amongst the 75 programs under review, only 25 programs were effective. While the low success rate might be in part attributed to weakly designed programs, it may also be due to poor program implementation and inability to implement the program as planned (2-4). As such, it is important to understand the quality of program implementation and whether the program has been implemented as intended. While outcome evaluation answers the question of whether a program works or not, process evaluation gives some clues to "why" an intervention program works and "how" it is delivered (5-7). Generally speaking, five aspects of program implementation are commonly focused upon, including "context", "reach", "dose delivered", "dose received" and "fidelity of intervention delivered" (8). While "context" refers to the conditions (such as settings) that affect the implementation of the program, "reach" is the proportion of the intended participants who actually join in the program. Besides, "dose delivered" refers to the amount of intended intervention that was actually delivered to the target audience whereas "dose received" means whether there was active engagement of the participants and their satisfaction with the intervention. Finally, "fidelity" refers to the quality of the implementation that was delivered in the intended manner.

There are research findings showing that low level of program fidelity is an important factor leading to program failure (9,10). In fact, interventions were found to be effective only when they were implemented with high levels of fidelity (11-13). According to Dane and Schneider (14), there are four key components of program fidelity. These included adherence (how well the major components of the program are implemented according to stated objectives), exposure (the extent to which the program is actually delivered to participants), quality of program delivery (the extent of the program is delivered in a quality manner) and participant responsiveness (degree of active engagement of the participants). Obviously, quality of program implementation is an important aspect of program implementation.

An integration of the literature on curricular-based positive youth development programs shows that quality of program implementation can be reflected by the following attributes of the program (15):

1. *Student interest*: whether the program can arouse the curiosity and capture the attention of the participants.
2. *Active involvement of students*: whether the program can engage the students and promote participation of the students.
3. *Classroom management*: whether classroom routines can be smoothly carried out and the intended activities can be successfully executed.
4. *Interactive delivery method*: whether two-way communication is present and the degree of interaction is high.

5. *Strategies to enhance the motivation of students*: whether varied learning strategies are used to motivate student learning.
6. *Positive feedback*: whether there is any use of praise and encouragement to promote student engagement and motivation.
7. *Familiarity of implementers with the students*: whether program implementers know the students.
8. *Reflective learning*: whether students are encouraged to reflect and think about their experiences so that deeper learning could be promoted.
9. *Program goal attainment*: whether the goals of the programs are attained.
10. *Time management*: whether class time is efficiently used.
11. *Familiarity of program implementers with the implementation materials*: whether the program implementers know the materials so that the messages are conveyed effectively to the students.

Under the New Undergraduate Curriculum at The Hong Kong Polytechnic University, a course entitled "Tomorrow's Leaders" was designed to fulfill the General University Requirements in the area of Leadership and Intrapersonal Development. A pilot course was conducted in the second term of 2010/11 academic year to test out the developed curriculum, with a total of 268 students in four classes participating in the course. Several evaluation mechanisms including objective outcome evaluation, post-course subjective outcome evaluation, post-lecture subjective outcome evaluation, process evaluation and qualitative evaluation were carried out (16-22). Overall speaking, the evaluation findings clearly suggest that the subject was able to promote the psychosocial competencies of the students.

To further test out the subject, a second piloting exercise was carried out in the first term of 2011/12 academic year. The topics covered in different lectures are presented in Table 1. Again, different forms of evaluation were conducted to examine the effectiveness of the subject. The purpose of the present study was to evaluate the subject via process evaluation. Two major research questions were asked in this study. (a) What was the overall implementation quality of the course entitled "Tomorrow's Leaders" at The Hong Kong Polytechnic University? (b) What were the correlates of program implementation quality and program success for this course?

METHODS

The proposed subject was piloted in the first term of 2011/12 academic year. The subject was offered to four classes, with a total of 195 students. In these classes, process evaluation was conducted in 19 lectures. Two observers were involved in the process and they were professionally trained social workers. During the observations, each observer completed a rating form covering program adherence and quality of program delivery.

Table 1. Summary of 14 lectures in the second piloting exercise

Lecture	Objectives	Content of Lecture	Example of activities
Lecture 1: Introduction and Self-Understanding	• To introduce the unique features and the outline of the course • To understand basic concepts and theories related to leadership and self-understanding • To examine the relationship between self-understanding and leadership • To enhance students' self-awareness and self-understanding abilities	• An overview of the course • Introduction to the concepts and models of leadership • An overview of the personal attributes of effective leaders • Role of self-understanding and interpersonal relationship qualities • Ways to promote self-development: a multilevel model	**Self-reflection exercise**: "Do I know myself?" **Purpose**: To help students to have a better understanding about their inner self • Distribute a worksheet to all students. • Ask students to write down 5 attributes or words that best describe themselves. • Ask students to share their views and feelings with the one who sit next to him/her. • Debrief after the exercise and highlight the importance of self-understanding.
Lecture 2: Personality	• To understand the definition, basic concepts, theories, and assessment related to personality • To summarize factors affecting the development of personality and its consequences • To examine personality and leadership • To help students explore ways to promote a mature personality that contributes to effective leadership	• Definition and major theories of personality: biological, humanist, psychoanalytic, trait and dispositional theories • Assessment of personality: five-factor model of personality • Personality and leadership: personality attributes conducive to successful leadership; contigency theory • Ways to promote a mature personality to achieve great leadership	**Group discussion**: "How well are my needs satisfied?" **Purpose**: To review and apply Maslow's hierarchy of needs theory in real settings • Ask students to evaluate their personality with reference to Maslow's hierarchy of needs. ○ Are my physical needs satisfied? ○ Am I a psychologically secure person? ○ Do I have a good social network? ○ Do I respect myself and love myself? ○ Am I self-actualizing? • Discuss in group regarding "do I respect and love myself?"
Lecture 3: Emotional Competence	• To introduce concepts and theories of emotional competence (EC) • To help students understand the antecedents and consequences of EC • To enhance students' awareness of EC • To examine the relationship between EC and leadership	• Awareness and understanding of EC • Theoretical framework for EC: emotional quotient (EQ), Saarni's 8 skills for EC • Role of EC in effective leadership: emotional management, empathy, self-awareness and good leadership • Strategies for emotion regulation	**Class activity**: "Emotion express" **Purpose**: To help students to express different emotions • Each group is given a worksheet. • Each group needs to write down a list of emotion words and to draw the corresponding faces (as many as possible in 4 minutes). • Do a little poll to see how many emotional words the students know
Lecture 4 Cognitive Competence	• To introduce the basic concepts and theories related to cognitive competence (CC)	• Understanding CC: definition of CC; a three-factor model of CC (what, how, and why); different types of thinking	**Class activity**: "Survival in the wilderness" **Purpose**: To enhance students' understanding of the role of different types of cognitive competence in problem-solving

Lecture	Objectives	Content of Lecture	Example of activities
	• To sum up factors affecting CC and its consequences • To examine the relationship between CC and leadership • To help students explore ways to promote CC	• Antecedents and consequences of CC • CC and effective leadership: metacognition and problem-solving • Ways to promote CC: cognitive training; learning; self-reflection	• Introduce the background of the game. • Ask students to work in groups to select 5 items in order to survive and list the reasons why they choose these items. • Ask students to reflect on the related CC.
Lecture 5: Resilience	• To introduce the basic concepts and theories on resilience (RE) • To help students understand the antecedents and consequences of RE • To examine the relationship between RE and leadership • To suggest a variety of ways to promote RE	• Understanding RE: definition and research on RE; components of RE • Importance of RE: stresses faced by adolescents, life adversities, coping with life stresses • Role of RE in effective leadership: characteristics of a resilient leader; positive psychological capital • Promote RE: proactive and reactive approaches	**Class activity**: "Star of resilience" **Purpose**: To learn from leaders who bounced back from adversity • Share resilient stories of four leaders with students. • Ask students to nominate one "Star of Resilience" from the four leaders or other leaders not being mentioned in the stories.
Lecture 6: Spirituality	• To introduce the definitions, basic concepts and theories related to spirituality (SP) • To summarize the antecedents and consequences of SP • To examine the relationship between SP and leadership • To explore ways to promote SP	• Definitions and theories of SP: connectedness to others; personal beliefs and values; meaning of life • Development of spirituality: factors affecting SP; SP and mental health • Role of spirituality in effective leadership • Strategies to promote SP: reflect on spiritual questions and experiences	**Self-reflection & sharing**: "Share your spirituality" **Purpose**: To help students reflect on their own meaning of life and the importance of spirituality • Invite students to reflect on: ○ How do you connect with others? ○ What are the most important personal beliefs and values in your life? ○ What is the meaning of your life?
Lecture 7: Ethics and Morality	• To introduce the concepts and theories related to ethics and morality (EM) • To help students understand the antecedents and consequences of EM • To examine the relationship between EM and leadership • To provide ways to promote morality and ethical leadership	• Understanding EM: definitions of ethics and morality; ten universal values for ethical behavior • Frameworks for moral judgment: Kohlberg's model of moral development; moral judgment competence; ethical decision-making • EM and leadership: ethical leadership; role of morality in effective leadership • Ways to promote EM	**Group discussion**: "What should Heinz do?" **Purpose**: To help students understand their moral judgment competence by presenting a hypothetical dilemma • Share the story of "Heinz" with the whole class. • Students are divided into 8 groups and asked to discuss the following questions: ○ Should Heinz steal the drug for his wife? ○ Why or why not?

Table 1. (Continued)

Lecture	Objectives	Content of Lecture	Example of activities
Lecture 8: Social Competence	• To understand definition, theories and concepts of social competence (SC) • To summarize the antecedents and consequences of SC • To examine the relationship between SC and leadership • To explore ways to promote SC	• Definitions and theories of SC; basic social competence skills • Antecedents and consequences of SC. • SC and leadership: role of self-awareness, self-management, social awareness, relationship management, empathy in effective leadership • Ways to promote SC: tips of developing SC; avoidance of egocentrism	**Warm-up acitivity**: "Story of a Master's degree holder" **Purpose**: To introduce the concept of SC by watching a video clip • Play the video clip about a Master's degree holder failing more than 200 job interviews and having to live on social welfare. • Ask students to discuss the problems related to social competence of the character in the video.
Lecture 9: Positive and Healthy Identity	• To introduce concepts and theories related to positive identity (PI) • To outline the antecedents and consequences of having PI • To discuss the role of PI in leadership • To help students explore ways to promote the development of PI	• Basic concepts and theories of self-identity: a hierarchical model of self-concept • Antecedents and consequences of PI • PI and leadership: a model of authentic leadership and followership • Ways to promote PI: self-evaluation; self-efficacy; self-acceptance; authentic living	**Class acitivity**: "The image of a successful leader" **Purpose**: To encourage students to discuss the attributes of a successful leader and reflect on their own identity • Based on a word list, students are asked to identify three most important attributes for a successful leader and write them down on the labels. • Each group will design a poster by using the hand-on materials and putting the labels on the poster.
Lecture 10: Interpersonal Communication	• To introduce the concepts and theories of interpersonal communication (IC) • To understand factors that influence IC and its consequences • To highlight the importance of IC in leadership • To recommend ways to promote good IC	• Definitions and theories of IC:; seven principles of IC • Antecedents and consequences of IC: skills and blocks of IC; importance of IC in different areas • IC and leadership: role of IC in effective leadership • Ways to promote IC: make your IC more effective, appropriate, ethical, and empathic	**Role play acitivity**: "The leader I like most!" **Purpose**: To let students reflect on different communication style of leaders • Brief the scenario to the class. • In each group, four students act as leaders, one as follower, and the others as observers. • Each leader is assigned one communication style, and gives the follower a verbal response according to the style. • Students discuss in groups which response is the most effective.
Lecture 11: Interpersonal conflict and team building	• To introduce the concept of interpersonal conflict and team building • To understand the relationship between interpersonal conflicts, team building and effective leadership	• Definitions and consequences of interpersonal conflict • Interpersonal conflict and leadership: 5 conflict-handling modes; role of conflict resolution in leadership	**Open discussion**: "Factors leading to conflicts" **Purpose**: To help students identify the causes or factors of interpersonal conflicts • Distribute Worksheet 1 (a list of factors) to students. • Ask students to decide which factors commonly lead to their conflicts with others.

Lecture	Objectives	Content of Lecture	Example of activities
	• To explore ways to manage interpersonal conflicts and develop team building	• Team building: manage conflict in teamwork; relationship building and effective leadership; assertiveness • Ways to promote team building	• Invite 2-3 students to share their thoughts. • Warp-up by showing components of conflict and common factors of interpersonal conflicts
Lecture 12: Integrity, Responsibility, and Egocentrism	• To introduce the concepts of integrity, responsibility, and egocentrism • To understand factors that influence integrity, responsibility, and egocentrism and their consequences • To highlight the importance of integrity, responsibility and egocentrism in leadership	• Theories and definitions of integrity, responsibility, and egocentrism • Consequences of integrity, responsibility, and egocentrism • Personal integrity and sense of responsibility in effective leaders; egocentricism and authenticity in university students	**Warm-up acitivity**: "Do you bring your unique peanut?" **Purpose**: To introduce the importance of resonsibility & integrity • Ask students to take out the peanut assigned to them last lecture. • See how many students can show the peanut; students who keep the peanut in a good shape will be awarded a small gift.
Lecture 13: Integrity, responsibility, and Egocentrism	• To introduce the concepts and theories of self-leadership • To understand relationship between self-leadership and mental health • To highlight the importance of self-leadership • To recommend ways to promote self-leadership	• Theories and definitions of self-leadership (SL) • SL and mental health: a model of SL and performance; relationship between SL and mental health • SL and effective leadership: SL within organization • Ways to promote SL	**Class acitivity**: "How well are you leading yourself?" **Purpose**: To help students aware of their self-leadership level through a self-administered questionnaire • Distribute Worksheet 1 (a self-leadership questionnaire) to all students. • Students are asked to finish the questionnaire and calculate the total scores they obtained.
Lecture 14: Summary and evaluation	• To summarize the course • To help students reflect on their experiences in this course	• A review of quality of effective leaders • A summary of the characteristics, students' comments, and evaluative findings of the course • Students' individual and group reflection	**Personal reflection**: "I reflect, therefore I exist." **Purpose**: To help student reflect on their experiences about this course • Ask students to write down descriptors and metaphors about the course; have group sharing on the related materials.

The observers evaluated the quality of delivery in terms of 13 areas including student interest, student participation and involvement, classroom control, use of interactive delivery method, use of strategies to enhance student motivation, use of positive and supportive feedbacks, instructors' familiarity with the students, opportunity for reflection, degree of achievement of the objectives, time management, quality of preparation, overall implementation quality, and success of implementation. For program adherence, the observers rated the degree of adherence and recorded the time used to implement the unit. This observation form was used in the first piloting exercise and it has been used in several process evaluation studies in Hong Kong (23-26). The observers were required not to discuss with each other during the process so that they would be "blind" to the ratings of the partner when they completed the observation forms.

Table 2. Inter-rater agreement between Rater 1 and Rater 2 on the observation items and program adherence

Item	Correlation between Rater 1 and Rater 2
1. How interested were the students in this lecture?	**0.906** **
2. To what extent did the students participate in lecture activities?	**0.789** **
3. To what extent was the lecture well managed?	**0.678** *
4. How interactive was the delivery method?	**0.722** ***
5. To what extent motivating strategies were used to motivate the students?	**0.622** *
6. How often were positive and supportive feedbacks elicited from the students?	**0.920** **
7. To what extent did the lecturer know the students?	**0.726** **
8. To what extent was reflection encouraged?	**0.734** **
9. To what extent were the objectives achieved?	**0.826** **
10. How well was the time managed?	**0.878** **
11. How well was the lecture prepared?	**0.900** **
12. Overall speaking, do you think the quality of implementation of this lecture was high?	**1.000** **
13. Overall speaking, do you think the implementation of the subject was successful?	**1.000** **
14. Program adherence	**0.884** **

Note: ***p<.001; **p<.01; *p<.05.

FINDINGS

For every lecture, the mean ratings for each item by the two independent observers were first calculated. To obtain an overall picture, scores for each item across all lectures were further averaged. The 13-item process evaluation scale was found to be internally consistent (Cronbach's alpha = 0.81, mean inter-item correlation = 0.25). As shown in Table 2, Pearson correlation analyses also showed that inter-rater reliability was very high. Regarding the ratings for the quality of delivery, results in Table 3 and Table 4 revealed that the quality of implementation as assessed by the two observers was generally high. In other words, both observers regarded the program implementation as successful. In particular, the average overall adherence to the developed curriculum was 94.9%, indicating very high program fidelity.

Table 3. Perception of program implementation quality based on the rating scale

Item	Rater 1: Percentage of positive responses (5-7)[a]	Rater 2: Percentage of positive responses (5-7)[a]	Mean Percentage of positive responses across raters (5-7)[a]
1. How interested were the students in this lecture?	**89.5%**	**100%**	**94.8%**
2. To what extent did the students participate in lecture activities?	**100%**	**100%**	**100%**
3. To what extent was the lecture well managed?	**100%**	**100%**	**100%**
4. How interactive was the delivery method?	**100%**	**100%**	**100%**
5. To what extent motivating strategies were used to motivate the students?	**94.7%**	**100%**	**97.4%**
6. How often were positive and supportive feedbacks elicited from the students?	**100%**	**100%**	**100%**
7. To what extent did the lecturer know the students?	**84.2%**	**84.2%**	**84.2%**
8. To what extent was reflection encouraged?	**94.7%**	**100%**	**97.4%**
9. To what extent were the objectives achieved?	**100%**	**100%**	**100%**
10. How well was the time managed?	**89.5%**	**94.7%**	**92.1%**
11. How well was the lecture prepared?	**89.5%**	**89.5%**	**89.5%**
12. Overall speaking, do you think the quality of implementation of this lecture was high?	**100%**	**100%**	**100%**
13. Overall speaking, do you think the implementation of the subject was successful?	**100%**	**100%**	**100%**

Note: [a] In Item 1 to Item 13, a 7-point (1-7) rating scale is used, with a higher score indicating better implementation quality. Specifically, 1, 2 and 3 represent for negative responses; 4 represents for neutral response; and 5, 6, and 7 represent for positive responses.

Table 4. Descriptive findings on the different dimensions of process evaluation

Item and adherence	Mean rating by Rater 1 across 19 lectures under observation	Mean rating by Rater 2 across 19 lectures under observation	Overall Mean Rating
1. Student Interest	5.58	5.63	5.61
2. Student participation and involvement	6.11	5.95	6.03
3. Classroom management	5.47	5.58	5.53
4. Interactive delivery method	5.89	5.79	5.84
5. Strategies to enhance student motivation	5.79	5.74	5.76
6. Use of positive and supportive feedbacks	5.42	5.32	5.37
7. Lecturer's familiarity with the students	5.05	5.21	5.13
8. Opportunities for reflection	5.58	5.53	5.55
9. Achievement of lecture objectives	6.05	5.79	5.92
10. Time management	5.53	5.58	5.84
11. Lecture preparation	6.00	5.68	5.74
12. Overall implementation quality	5.74	5.74	5.79
13. Success of implementation	5.79	5.79	5.55
Adherence	95.16	94.63	94.90

Note: In Item 1 to Item 13, a 7-point (1-7) rating scale is used, with a higher score indicating better implementation quality.

Table 5. Correlation between different dimensions of program implementation and adherence and overall program implementation quality and success

Measures	Overall implementation quality	Overall implementation success
1. Student Interest	.39 ns	.33 ns
2. Student participation and involvement	.25 ns	.26 ns
3. Classroom management	.69 **	.62 **
4. Interactive delivery method	.29 ns	.33 ns
5. Strategies to enhance student motivation	.04 ns	.15 ns
6. Use of positive and supportive feedbacks	.35 ns	.30 ns
7. Lecturer's familiarity with the students	.02 ns	.00 ns
8. Opportunities for reflection	.32 ns	.39 ns
9. Achievement of lecture objectives	.83 **	.73 **
10. Time management	.77 **	.74 **
11. Lecture preparation	.76 **	.81 **
12. Adherence	.36 ns	.29 ns

Note: $^{**}p<.01$; $^{*}p<.05$; ns = non-significant.

Concerning correlates of program implementation quality and program success, results showed that classroom management, time management, achievement of objectives and lecture preparation were significant correlates (see Table 5). In view of the small sample size, the findings could be regarded as robust.

DISCUSSION

In this study, program adherence and quality of implementation of a course entitled "Tomorrow's Leaders" offered at The Hong Kong Polytechnic University were examined via systematic observations of 19 lectures delivered in four classes of students in the second piloting exercise. Regarding reliability of the findings, two observations can be highlighted from the present study. First, despite the small number of observations (N = 19 lectures), the 13-item rating scale for process evaluation was found to be internally consistent. Second, inter-rater reliability was very encouraging, suggesting that there is a high level of agreement amongst the two raters. The high level of agreement may be due to the fact that only two raters were employed in this study.

The findings based on descriptive statistics showed two phenomena. First, the average level of adherence to the teaching materials was on the high side. The findings suggest that there was no apparent need to change the curriculum. This observation is very important if a large number of classes are involved. Second, the two observers perceived that the objectives of the units implemented could be achieved and the overall quality of implementation was high with reference to the different aspects of the subject, including students' interest and involvement, classroom management, interactive teaching strategies used by the instructors, and students' reflection in the course. Nevertheless, although the findings are very encouraging, there were two areas that had "relatively lower" mean scores. The first area was the use of positive and supportive feedbacks. As the demand for interactive teaching was quite high for this course and the Chinese teachers are usually didactic in their teaching, these attributes may contribute to the relatively "lower" scores. Second, it was found that teacher's familiarity with the student was relatively low. This is understandable because there were around 50 students in each class. As such, the teachers might find it difficult to be familiar with the students, hence contributing to the observed phenomenon.

Regarding the correlates of program implementation quality and success, results showed that classroom management, time management, achievement of objectives were significant correlates of overall implementation quality and success. While this observation is in line with the research findings in the first piloting exercise, it is interesting to note that other aspects were not significantly correlated with overall program implementation quality and success in this study. There are two possible explanations for this finding. First, the inconsistency may be due to the small sample size in both studies. Second, the inconsistency may be due to the employment of different raters in the two studies. While several raters were involved in Study 1, two raters were consistently employed in Study 2. As the findings on the correlates of program implementation quality and success are not conclusive, future studies should be carried out to clarify this issue. Furthermore, as there are research findings showing that active engagement of participants is a critical factor for the program implementation process (27,28), there is a need to explore this aspect further.

The present study clearly replicated and extended the findings in the first piloting exercise. However, there are several limitations of the study. First, as only 19 lectures were observed, it would be desirable to include more lectures for observations in future. Second, besides the quality of implementation dimensions adopted in this study, additional dimensions such as the degree of involvement and care of the instructor as well as the learning opportunities in the subject should be included. Third, generalization of the present findings to other settings should proceed with caution because of the small sample size involved. Despite these limitations, in conjunction with previous research findings, the present findings strongly suggest that the quality of implementation of "Tomorrow's Leaders" was high and the course was able to promote psychosocial competencies in the students taking this course.

ACKNOWLEDGMENTS

This work and the course on "Tomorrow's Leaders" are financially supported by The Hong Kong Polytechnic University. Members of the Curriculum Development Team include Daniel T.L. Shek, Y.H. Chui, S.W. Lit, Yida Y.H. Chung, Sowa S.W. Ngai, Yammy L.Y. Chak, P.F. Tsui, Cecilia M.S. Ma, Lu Yu and Moon Y.M. Law. This chapter has been published as a paper in the International Journal on Disability and Human Development 2013;12(2). Permission has been obtained from De Gruyter to re-publish in this modified form.

REFERENCES

[1] Catalano RF, Berglund ML, Ryan JA, Lonczak HS, Hawkins JD. Positive youth development in the United States: research findings on evaluations of positive youth development programs. Prev Treat 2002;5:1-111.

[2] Drug Strategies. Save schools, safe students: a guide to violence prevention strategies. Washington, DC: Drug Strategies, 1998.
[3] Durlak JA, Wells AM. Evaluation of indicated preventive intervention (secondary prevention) mental health programs for children and adolescents. Am J Commun Psychol 1998;26:775-802.
[4] Tobler NS. Drug prevention programs can work: research findings. J Addict Dis 1992;11:1-28.
[5] Dusenbury L, Branningan R, Falco M, Hansen WB. A review of research on fidelity of implementation: implications for drug abuse prevention in school settings. Health Educ Res 2003;18:237-56.
[6] Yeaton WH, Sechrest L. Critical dimensions in the choice and maintenance of successful treatment: strength, integrity and effectiveness. J Consul Clin Psychol 1981;49:156-67.
[7] McCreary LL, Koponda CP, Kafulafula UK, Ngalande RC, Kumbani LC, Jere DL, Norr JL, Norr KF. Process evaluation of HIV prevention peer groups in Malawi: a look inside the black box. Health Educ Res 2010;25(6):965-78.
[8] Linnan L, Steckler A. Process evaluation for public health interventions and research: an overview. In: Stecker A, Linnan L, editors. Process evaluation for public health interventions and research. San Francisco, CA: Jossey-Bass, 2001:1-23.
[9] Durlak JA, DuPre EP. Implementation matters: a review of research on the influence of implementation on program outcomes and the factors affecting implementation. Am J Commun Psychol 2008;41:327-50.
[10] Lipsey M. The primary factors that characterize effective interventions with juvenile offenders: a meta-analytic overview. Vict Offender 2009;4:124-47.
[11] Kam CM, Greenberg MT, Walls CT. Examining the role of implementation quality in school-based prevention using the paths curriculum: promoting alternative thinking skills curriculum. Prev Sci 2003;4:55-63.
[12] Mihalic S, Fagan A, Argamaso S. Implementing the life-skills training drug prevention program: factors related to implementation fidelity. Implem Sci 2008;3:5-21.
[13] Mihalic S. The importance of implementation fidelity. Emot Behav Disord Youth 2004;4:83-105.
[14] Dane AV, Schneider BH. Program integrity in primary and early secondary prevention: are implementation effects out of control? Clin Psychol Rev 1998;18:23-4.
[15] Law BMF, Shek DTL. Process evaluation of a positive youth development program in Hong Kong based on different cohorts. ScientificWorldJournal 2012, Article ID 736730, 9 pages. DOI: 10.1100/2012/736730.
[16] Shek DTL, Sun RCF. Promoting psychosocial competencies in university students: evaluation based on a one group pretest-posttest design. Int J Disabil Hum Dev 2012;11:229-34.
[17] Shek DTL, Sun RCF. Promoting leadership and intrapersonal competence in university students: what can we learn from Hong Kong? Int J Disabil Hum Dev 2012;11:221-28..
[18] Shek DTL, Sun RCF. Process evaluation of a positive youth development course in a university setting in Hong Kong. Int J Disabil Hum Dev 2012;11:235-41..
[19] Shek DTL, Sun RCF. Qualitative evaluation of a positive youth development course in a university setting in Hong Kong. Int J Disabil Hum Dev 2012;11:243-48.
[20] Shek DTL, Sun RCF. Focus group evaluation of a positive youth development course in a university in Hong Kong. Int J Disabil Hum Dev 2012;11:249-54.
[21] Shek DTL. Postlecture evaluation of a positive youth development subject for university students in Hong Kong. ScientificWorldJournal 2012, Article ID 934679, 8 pages.DOI:10.1100/2012/934679.
[22] Shek DTL. Reflective journals of students taking a positive youth development course in a university context in Hong Kong. ScientificWorldJournal 2012, Article ID 131560, 8 pages. DOI: 10.1100/2012/131560.
[23] Shek DTL, Yu L. Longitudinal impact of the Project P.A.T.H.S. on adolescent risk behavior: what happened after five years? ScientificWorldJournal 2012, Article ID 316029, 13 pages. DOI: 10.1100/2012/316029.
[24] Sun RCF, Shek DTL. Positive youth development, life satisfaction and problem behavior among Chinese adolescents in Hong Kong: a replication. Soc Indic Res 2012;105:541-59.

[25] Shek DTL. Qualitative evaluation of Project P.A.T.H.S. in Hong Kong: focus groups based on Secondary 3 program implementers. Int J Disabil Hum Dev 2012;24:245-52.

[26] Shek DTL, Ma CMS, Kan VWM. Subjective outcome evaluation of Project P.A.T.H.S. based on different cohorts of students. Int J Disabil Hum Dev 2011;10:227-34.

[27] Byrnes HF, Miller BA, Aalborg AE, Plasencia AV, Keagy CD. Implementation fidelity in adolescent family-based prevention programs: relationship to family engagement. Health Educ Res 2010;25: 531-41.

[28] Spoth R, Redmond C. Research on family engagement in preventive interventions: toward improved use of scientific findings in primary prevention practice. J Prim Prev 2000;21:267-84.

In: Chinese Adolescent Development ISBN: 978-1-62618-622-4
Editors: Daniel TL Shek, Rachel CF Sun, Joav Merrick © 2013 Nova Science Publishers, Inc.

Chapter 11

REFLECTIONS OF CHINESE STUDENTS ON A UNIVERSITY SUBJECT ON LEADERSHIP AND INTRAPERSONAL DEVELOPMENT

Daniel TL Shek [*,1,2,3,4,5] ***and Luana YK Tung*** [1]

[1]Department of Applied Social Sciences,
The Hong Kong Polytechnic University, Hong Kong, PRC
[2] Centre for Innovative Programmes for Adolescents and Families The Hong Kong Polytechnic University, Hong Kong, PRC
[3]Kiang Wu Nursing College of Macau, Macau, PRC
[4]Department of Social Work, East China Normal University, Shanghai, PRC
[5]Division of Adolescent Medicine, Department of Pediatrics,
Kentucky Children's Hospital, University of Kentucky College of Medicine,
Lexington, Kentucky, US

ABSTRACT

To examine the effectiveness of a university subject (Tomorrow's Leaders) which attempts to promote holistic development in students, students were invited to write personal reflections about the subject. Based on the reflections of 104 students, data were separately rated by two independent raters using a standardized rating form. Intra-rater and inter-rater reliability analyses revealed that the coding of reflections was reliable. Results showed that the informants were generally positive about the subject and lecturers and they perceived that the subject promoted their overall development in different domains. Exemplar cases were highlighted in this chapter.

[*] Correspondence: Professor Daniel TL Shek, PhD, FHKPS, BBS, JP, Chair Professor of Applied Social Sciences, Faculty of Health and Social Sciences, Department of Applied Social Sciences, The Hong Kong Polytechnic University, Room HJ407, Core H, Hunghom, Hong Kong. E-mail: daniel.shek@polyu.edu.hk

INTRODUCTION

The dominant mode of research in human development is quantitative research which is rooted in empiricism. There are several unique features of quantitative research, including emphasis on techniques and procedures involving sensory experiences (i.e., seeing is believing), drawing representative samples, development of precise instruments, treating experimental control and experimental designs as superior forms of research, reliance on rigorous statistical analyses involving hypotheses testing, and focusing on hypothetical-deductive models. According to Neuman and Kreuger (1), positivistic social science is a research paradigm in which deductive logic is combined with precise empirical observations, with the aims of discovering and confirming probabilistic causal laws and predicting human and social activity patterns. Positivistic scientists believe that scientists can discover "preexisting regularities" in social and physical reality just like taking photographs. Besides, they believe that scientific explanations are nomothetic universal laws which are generalizable across spatial and historical contexts. To determine the truth, scientists use stringent empirical methods to test hypotheses. In the process, logical thinking is valued and values and feelings of the scientists should be minimized or eliminated (2).

Nevertheless, there are growing criticisms about the quantitative approach in human development research (3-7). First, focus on experimental approach and "rigorous" research methods has been regarded as ignoring the social contexts in which human behavior occurs (i.e., context stripping). Second, while it is assumed that behavior or human response has a single meaning in positivistic research, it is argued that there can be multiple meanings of human behavior, thus making the role of interpretations important. Third, the dualist assumption of independence of theories and observations is doubtful because of the theory-ladenness of facts. Fourth, as values and evidence are interdependent, it is impossible to have total objectivity. This point is highlighted in the work of Thomas Kuhn that even science has its tradition and there were changing emphases throughout history. Finally, as the inquirers may influence the observed and there is non-existence of impartial observers, the interactive nature of scientific inquiry cannot be totally objective (2).

In response to the inadequacies of the quantitative approach to understand human development, there is a call for the use of qualitative research. Although there are many philosophical roots of qualitative inquiries, the qualitative approach is closely linked to interpretivism. In interpretive research, researchers analyze socially meaningful actions normally through direct and detailed observations and in-depth understanding of people in their natural settings. For qualitative researchers, social reality is based on people's definition and meaning. The social reality can be a subjectively constructed world (phenomenology) or socially constituted reality (social constructionism). In contrast to the positivistic notion that human beings are passive reactors to external stimulation, interpretive researchers regard human beings as meaning generating agents who are capable of reflection. In addition, description and interpretation are the fundamental tasks of researchers who seek to identify idiographic understanding (individual uniqueness) mainly through inductive analyses. By making "thick description", a novel or story is similar to a mathematical proof or geographical map which can reveal the meanings and rules of living used by people in their daily lives. Furthermore, it is argued that "facts" are fluid and embedded within a meaning system; hence they are not impartial, objective, or neutral. In the realm of evaluation, these two dominant approaches to research have been utilized by evaluators (3-7).

This chapter attempts to report evaluation findings on a university subject on leadership and intrapersonal development. Under the New Undergraduate Curriculum implemented in 2012, a credit-bearing subject entitled “Tomorrow’s Leaders” was developed at The Hong Kong Polytechnic University.

This subject is intended to help students understand positive youth development constructs, including self-understanding, personality, emotional competence, cognitive competence, resilience, spirituality, social competence, moral competence, positive identity, interpersonal communication, conflict resolution, team building, and relationship building. Different teaching methods, including brief lectures, experiential learning activities, group presentations, and individual assignments are used to promote the psychosocial competencies of the students. It is expected that students will be able to understand and integrate theories, research, and concepts on the basic qualities (particularly intrapersonal and interpersonal qualities) of effective leaders, develop self-awareness and understanding of oneself, acquire interpersonal skills, and develop self-reflection skills in their learning after taking this subject.

This subject was piloted in 2010/11 academic year. To understand the effectiveness of the subject, different evaluation strategies were employed, with very positive evaluation outcomes (8-14). To further refine the subject and to accumulate more teaching experience, the subject was piloted again in the first term of 2011/12 academic year.

As not much in-depth qualitative data were collected in the first piloting exercise, more qualitative data were collected in the second piloting exercise. In this study, students were invited to write personal reflections on their experiences of the subject. The cases collected were then subject to thematic coding. Exemplar cases are then shown to illustrate the effectiveness of the subject.

STUDY

In the first term of 2011/12 academic year, the subject “Tomorrow’s Leaders” was offered to 195 students in four classes. Toward the end of the subject, students were invited to write down some personal reflections about the subject.

The reflections could include their views about the subject matter, lectures, lecturers, benefits of the subject, changes after taking this subject, problems of the subject (if any), and overall personal reflections. Students could write in Chinese (around 400 words) or English (around 300 words) and they could hand in their reflections in hard copies or soft copies.

A total of 104 pieces of personal reflections were collected from the students. To enhance objectivity of the coding process, the data were coded and analyzed by two research staff using a standardized coding form (see Table 1). Using the form, the raters determined the tone of the reflections regarding the subject (e.g., relevant to university students), class (e.g., interactive), lecturer (e.g., caring), and benefits (e.g., promotion of resilience). In addition, an overall score ranging from 0-10 was given by each rater. To enhance the reliability of the coding of different aspects of the reflections, both intra- and inter-rater reliability tests were carried out. For intra-rater reliability, each rater re-coded 10 randomly selected cases. For inter-rater reliability, 10 cases from each rater were re-coded by another rater.

Table 1. Coding form for the personal reflection

Case Number: ______

Name of the Coder: ____________________________

Date of Coding: ________________________________

1. Comments on the Subject (e.g., content, topics, differences from other subjects)

a. Positive comments with no negative comments
b. Basically positive comments, but with some negative comments
c. Neutral descriptions (positive and negative comments are roughly equal)
d. Basically negative comments, but with some positive comments
e. Negative comments with no positive comments
f. Not applicable

2. Comments on the Class (e.g., interactive nature, fun)

a. Positive comments with no negative comments
b. Basically positive comments, but with some negative comments
c. Neutral descriptions (positive and negative comments are roughly equal)
d. Basically negative comments, but with some positive comments
e. Negative comments with no positive comments
f. Not applicable

3. Comments on the Teacher (e.g., care and teaching style)

a. Positive comments with no negative comments
b. Basically positive comments, but with some negative comments
c. Neutral descriptions (positive and negative comments are roughly equal)
d. Basically negative comments, but with some positive comments
e. Negative comments with no positive comments
f. Not applicable

4. Comments on the Benefits Gained (e.g., promotion of self-understanding)

a. Positive comments with no negative comments
b. Basically positive comments, but with some negative comments
c. Neutral descriptions (positive and negative comments are roughly equal)
d. Basically negative comments, but with some positive comments
e. Negative comments with no positive comments
f. Not applicable

Overall Tone (0 = Completely Negative; 10 = Completely Positive) = ______

FINDINGS

Aggregating the data from two raters, analyses showed that intra-rater reliability was high for subject (95%), class (100%), lecturer (95%), benefits (100%), and overall quality (85%). Similarly, analyses showed that inter-rater reliability was high for subject (95%), class (100%), lecturer (100%), benefits (100%), and overall quality (80%). Using 104 cases as the basis of analyses, Pearson correlation showed that there was high concordance of responses across the two independent raters for subject ($r=.84$, $p < .0001$), class ($r=.70$, $p < .0001$), lecturer ($r=1.0$, $p < .0001$), benefits ($r=.94$, $p < .0001$), and overall quality ($r=.92$, $p < .0001$).

Regarding the nature of reflections of the students, the findings were basically positive in nature. Generally speaking, the students had very positive evaluation of the subject, class, and teacher. Also, students perceived that there were many benefits gained from the subject and the overall evaluation of the subject was positive. With reference to the rating on the overall quality, 96.2% (Rater 1) and 94.2% (Rater 2) of the responses were in the positive direction. The findings can be seen in Table 2. Some exemplar cases can also be seen below:

- *Case 1:* When I had the first lesson of this class, I thought "Tomorrow's Leaders" was boring and it was all about theory. I even thought that it was not suitable for me to take this subject. However, after taking a few lessons, my view was changed. It is a useful course for me to enhance my personal development as it provided comprehensive topics about personal development and it promoted self-reflection. Some leadership skills have also been taught in the lesson in an interesting way.

  The most impressive topic for me is about ways of solving conflict. In fact, when I organized the orientation camp with my committee members, we had lots of quarrel. The bad time made me depressed and my emotion was out of control. When I learned in the lesson of conflict management, I always flashed back to the bad time and recognized that if I had solved the conflict in an appropriate way, it would not have been a bad time but a good time.
  I do appreciate that/how the lecturer taught the topics in a funny way. He always prepared videos, games or tests for us. This made the lessons so interesting and we learned in an effective way.

- *Case 2:* I learned a lot from this GE course. Although it's just a 2-credit course, we did enjoy and put much effort into it. We met new friends from different departments. We built up friendship and shared different points of view through discussion. In the lectures, the lecturer contributed his speech and he also allowed us to interact and communicate with classmates. We thought about and reflected on our own experiences of our lives. Now, "Tomorrow's Leaders" to me is not only a noun, but also something we could achieve in the future. I am glad that I have joined the course.

- *Case 3:* Actually, I quite enjoy the lectures of this subject. It is different from my core subject, which is only listening to the lecturer and memorizing all the Power Point, then exam. In this subject, there were many chances for us to reflect and to think more about ourselves. I don't know whether a leader should share more about himself/herself, as there were many discussion sessions in the lecture, encouraging students to speak, to voice their thoughts. In this subject "Tomorrow's Leaders", all the students may become leaders one day. The components of a leader, mentioned in each lecture, impressed me a lot and it will definitely benefit us when we face different types of leaders in the future.

Table 2. Ratings of Rater 1 and Rater 2 on the different aspects of the reflections submitted by the students

Rater 1	Mean (SD)
Subject	1.54 (0.93)
Class	1.02 (0.14)
Teacher	1.07 (0.37)
Benefits	1.09 (0.50)
Overall	8.55 (1.78)
Rater 2	
Subject	1.62 (1.01)
Class	1.02 (0.14)
Teacher	1.10 (0.56)
Benefits	1.09 (0.50)
Overall	8.49 (1.83)
Mean of Rater 1 and Rater 2	
Subject	1.58 (0.97)
Class	1.02 (0.14)
Teacher	1.09 (0.46)
Benefits	1.09 (0.50)
Overall	8.52 (1.81)

Apart from the teaching materials, the lecturer always encouraged us to voice the difficulties or thoughts on the lectures. He tried to enable us to have a better understanding on some components. He knew we love watching videos, so he showed a lot of videos related to the topic during the lectures so that the lectures became more attractive to us.

- *Case 4:* I think this course is useful since it taught us many essential elements that a leader should have. Every lecture, the lecturer organized many interactive activities which enhanced our memory. Moreover, the "pressure survey" impressed me most. It reflected my inner feelings. It made me aware that we should manage our pressure well. Also, I have developed self-reflection skills and acquired interpersonal skills which are very useful for my future development and growth. Finally, it is worthwhile for me to take this course. I am confident that I would be a leader soon.

  Moreover, the topic "Interpersonal Conflict and Team Building" impressed me a lot since it is easy for us to have conflicts when doing group projects. It is important for us to have good interpersonal relationship with group mates.

At the same time, we can handle conflicts well. Moreover, since I would be a social worker in the future, it is important for me to develop team building skills. I have acquired several ways to manage interpersonal conflicts and develop team building.

- *Case 5*: It is a valuable experience to study this subject. In the course of this subject, different activities, writings, and drawings enhanced my understanding about myself, including my strengths and weaknesses, which helped me improve my interpersonal skills. The topics taught in this subject are important to our daily living. For instance, we need emotional competence when our feeling is fluctuating; we need resilience when we are in a deadlock. Good interpersonal skill is a must for all of us nowadays when almost every one of us is holding a bachelor's degree. Our personality and how we deal with problems are more important than what we know.

  Through the activities in class, we reviewed our daily lives and we realized how we interacted with others. Thus, we learned about our personality. Also, the workload of this subject was low, such that actually this subject gave us a relaxed atmosphere to review our life and take a break in our schedule. It is really worthwhile to study and I think all the first year students of 3-3-4 should have their personality and mind prepared before they can further their study in university.

- *Case 6:* The lectures that I like most and are the most unforgettable to me are "Self-understanding" and "Resilience". For "Self-understanding", it provided a chance for us to rethink ourselves. I think it was a valuable opportunity for understanding our strengths and weaknesses. I know many people just keep judging others, but they may not know that they also have some problems. After understanding ourselves, it is a chance to let us accept and strive for change. Then, I believe that it will be easier to be a good leader and communicate with others after the change. This lecture definitely helped me!

  For "Resilience", I learned that we can convert difficulties into opportunities. The course taught us positive thinking and encouraged me to deal with the difficulties. Now in my mind, difficulties are just time to make decisions and time to prove that I have the ability to solve problems. This concept is useful for giving me power to deal with difficulties for the rest of my life. Last but not least, I liked the in-class activities, videos, and stories provided by the lecturers. They got me involved in the class and to cooperate with different people.

  When I attended other classes, there was no chance to interact with people, and no chance to meet new friends. But "Tomorrow's Leaders" has these opportunities! And also, it is valuable to meet people from different programs, such as engineering and social work. It is good to understand them and know more about their values, which are very different from mine. I would like to thank all the lecturers. Thank you for their teaching and thank you for their efforts.

- *Case 7:* During the GE subject registration period, I wondered if I could find a subject that was beneficial to my personal development. The subject "Tomorrow's Leaders" sounded interesting. Even though I believed that I might be a follower for the rest of my life (owing to my poor interpersonal skills), I was curious to know what qualities a good leader should have. Therefore, despite the discouragement from my friends, I considered this course the first priority. I think I have made the right choice for the reasons below.

  Firstly, the course strongly encouraged active participation. Having the courage to answer a question voluntarily means to participate actively, and to take the initiative is what a leader should do. To lead is to take the vanguard position. If you refuse to be the first one to go, will others follow you? The course provided us the chance to improve ourselves. I think I have grasped the chance to improve myself.

  Secondly, I think the teaching approach is impressive. Unlike conventional lectures, "Tomorrow's Leaders" is very dynamic. Various in-class activities such as games kept us from falling asleep. They stimulated us to participate more in the lecture and guided us to understand the lecture topics better. The lectures will definitely be dull without activities.

  Thirdly, leadership qualities are explained clearly. Not only do we have a theoretical framework on the qualities, but also we have real life examples and guidelines for us to develop these desirable traits. This means that the knowledge we obtained is applicable and realistic. The message is clear: you can make a change if you want to.

  To conclude, the course inspired me in various aspects, namely personal growth, interpersonal interaction and most importantly, how to be a good leader. These are not obtainable from the subjects in my major. It is my pleasure to take this course.

- *Case 8*: This course, "Tomorrow's Leaders", was very different from what I have taken in my major, Marketing. In my major, there are only lectures and tutorials. After the lecturers finished what they wanted to say, they left. Interactions were seldom seen. But in "Tomorrow's Leaders", there were many interactions which shocked me at the very beginning. Nearly everyone had to share what they think and feel during lessons. I was not used to this format of having lessons as I had never encountered it. But eventually, I started to adapt to this format and started to speak out in the lessons (although I am still a bit embarrassed). This is something I could never have encountered if I hadn't taken this course. Also, the most interesting part was the worksheet. At first, I thought the worksheet was just like homework in primary school. A bit weird. But later, I found that these few pieces of paper could help me find my truth and know about myself. I had the deepest feeling when I was filling the worksheet about my strengths, weaknesses, and ideal-self. I thought a lot. I would like to find out the answers. Fortunately, I found them, more than the worksheet required. I'm not sure if I'll become a good leader after taking the course, but I am sure I know more about myself. That's the first step to being a good leader, I think.

Discussion

According to Shek, there are few credit-bearing subjects on positive youth development designed for university students (15-16). Utilizing theories and research in positive youth development, a course entitled "Tomorrow's Leaders" was developed at The Hong Kong Polytechnic University. Besides implementing the subject, systematic evaluation was carried out. In contrast to quantitative methodology which focuses on numbers and statistical analyses, qualitative findings based on personal reflections were collected and analyzed in the present study. To overcome the problem of subjectivity in qualitative evaluation, both intra-rater and inter-rater reliability tests were carried out. The related findings clearly showed that both intra-rater and inter-rater reliability of the coding tasks were on the high side.

The findings based on the rating data revealed two observations. First, the course, class, and lecturer were perceived in a positive manner by the students. Using overall quality as the criteria, the ratings were on the high side; over 94% of the ratings were positive responses. Second, students generally perceived the benefits of taking this subject. Taken as a whole, the quantitative findings are consistent with the themes of the case studies. In conjunction with the evaluation findings based on post-lecture subjective outcome evaluation, post-course subjective outcome evaluation, and process evaluation, the present findings suggest that this subject was able to promote the development of the psychosocial competencies in students taking "Tomorrow's Leaders" (8-14).

As a qualitative evaluation study, it is important to watch out for alternative explanations in qualitative research (17).

First, the positive evaluation findings may be due to demand characteristics. However, this explanation is not likely because students were encouraged to express their views freely, and negative views were in fact recorded. In addition, the students wrote the reflections in an anonymous manner. Second, although it can be argued that the favourable findings were due to ideological biases of the author, several safeguards (e.g., intra- and inter-rater reliability as well as disciplined data analyses and interpretations) were used to reduce biases in the data collection and analysis process. Actually, the author was not involved in the data collection and coding process.

It is noteworthy that there are several limitations of the study. First, as the data were collected from only 104 students, there is a need to replicate the findings. Second, because students participated in the study in a voluntary manner, there is a need to understand why other students did not participate in the study. Third, besides personal reflections, more interactive forms of qualitative evaluation strategies such as in-depth individual interviews would enable the researchers to understand the inner worlds and subjective experiences of the students.

Despite the aforementioned limitations, the current study provides additional qualitative evaluation findings that support the positive nature of "Tomorrow's Leaders" and further confirm its effectiveness in promoting holistic youth development among Chinese university students in Hong Kong. Furthermore, it underscores the utility of the positive youth development approach in promoting holistic development of university students (18-23).

Acknowledgments

The development of the course titled "Tomorrow's Leaders" and the evaluation study were financially supported by The Hong Kong Polytechnic University via the Teaching Development Grant and the funding for the 3-3-4 new curriculum. We would also like to thank the Wofoo Foundation for the establishment of several scholarships for those outstanding students taking the course. This chapter has been published as a paper in the International Journal on Disability and Human Development, 2013;12(2). Permission has been obtained from De Gruyter to re-publish in this modified form.

References

[1] Neuman WL, Kreuger LW. Social work research methods: qualitative and quantitative approaches. Boston: Allyn Bacon, 2003.
[2] Leung JYT, Shek DTL. Quantitative and qualitative approaches in the study of poverty and adolescent development: separation or integration? Int J Adolesc Med Health 2011;23(2):115-21.
[3] Denzin NK, Lincoln YS. The Sage handbook of qualitative research. Thousands Oaks, CA: Sage, 2011.
[4] Creswell JW. Research design: qualitative, quantitative and mixed methods approaches. Thousand Oaks, CA: Sage, 2009.
[5] Burke J, Christensen L. Educational research: quantitative, qualitative, and mixed approaches. Los Angeles, CA: Sage, 2012.
[6] Posavac EJ. Program evaluation: methods and case studies. Boston, MA: Prentice Hall, 2011.
[7] Mertens DM. Research and evaluation in education and psychology: integrating diversity with quantitative, qualitative, and mixed methods. Thousand Oaks, CA: Sage, 2010.
[8] Shek DTL, Sun RCF. Promoting psychosocial competencies in university students: evaluation based on a one group pretest-posttest design. Int J Disabil Hum Dev 2012;11:229-34.
[9] Shek DTL, Sun RCF. Promoting leadership and intrapersonal competence in university students: what can we learn from Hong Kong? Int J Disabil Hum Dev 2012;11:221-8.
[10] Shek DTL, Sun RCF. Process evaluation of a positive youth development course in a university setting in Hong Kong. Int J Disabil Hum Dev 2012;11:235-42.
[11] Shek DTL, Sun RCF. Qualitative evaluation of a positive youth development course in a university setting in Hong Kong. Int J Disabil Hum Dev 2012;11:243-8.
[12] Shek DTL, Sun RCF. Focus group evaluation of a positive youth development course in a university in Hong Kong. Int J Disabil Hum Dev 2012;11:249-54.
[13] Shek DTL. Post-lecture evaluation of a positive youth development subject for university students in Hong Kong. ScientificWorldJournal 2012, Article ID 934679, 8 pages. DOI: 10.1100/2012/934679.
[14] Shek DTL, Wu FKY. Reflective journals of students taking a positive youth development course in a university context in Hong Kong. ScientificWorldJournal2012, Article ID 131560, 8 pages. DOI: 10.1100/2012/131560.
[15] Shek DTL. Nurturing holistic development of university students in Hong Kong: where are we and where should we go? ScientificWorldJournal 2010;10:563-75.
[16] Shek DTL, Wong KK. Do adolescent developmental issues disappear overnight? Reflections about holistic development in university students. ScientificWorldJournal 2011;11:353-61.
[17] Shek DTL, Tang V, Han XY. Quality of qualitative evaluation studies in the social work literature: evidence that constitutes a wakeup call. Res Soc Work Pract 2005;15:180-94.
[18] Shek DTL. Quality of life research: responses to emerging issues in a changing world. Soc Indic Res 2011;100(3):371-4.
[19] Shek DTL, Ma CMS, Tang CYP. Predictors of subjective outcome evaluation findings in a positive youth development program in Hong Kong. Int J Disabil Hum Dev 2011;10:249-55.

[20] Shek DTL, Sun RCF, Merrick J. Training programs and implementation process of positive youth development programs. Int J Adolesc Med Health 2011;23:303-4.

[21] Shek DTL, Ma HK, Sun RCF. A brief overview of adolescent developmental problems in Hong Kong. ScientificWorldJournal 2011;11:2243-56.

[22] Shek DTL, Ma HK, Sun RCF. Development of a new curriculum in a positive youth development program: the Project P.A.T.H.S. in Hong Kong. ScientificWorldJournal 2011;11:2207-18.

[23] Sun RCF, Shek DTL. Positive youth development, life satisfaction and problem behaviour among Chinese adolescents in Hong Kong: a replication. Soc Indic Res 2012;105:541-59.

In: Chinese Adolescent Development ISBN: 978-1-62618-622-4
Editors: Daniel TL Shek, Rachel CF Sun, Joav Merrick © 2013 Nova Science Publishers, Inc.

Chapter 12

OBJECTIVE OUTCOME EVALUATION OF A LEADERSHIP AND INTRAPERSONAL DEVELOPMENT SUBJECT FOR UNIVERSITY STUDENTS

Daniel TL Shek**[*,1,2,3,4,5]**, Rachel CF Sun**[6]**,
***Teresa BK Tsien-Wong**[1]**, Chung Tai Cheng**[1]*
***and Hai Rong Yan**[1]*

[1]Department of Applied Social Sciences, The Hong Kong Polytechnic University, Hong Kong, PRC
[2]Centre for Innovative Programmes for Adolescents and Families, The Hong Kong Polytechnic University, Hong Kong, PRC
[3]Kiang Wu Nursing College of Macau, Macau, PRC
[4]Department of Social Work, East China Normal University, Shanghai, PRC
[5]Division of Adolescent Medicine, Department of Pediatrics, Kentucky Children's Hospital, University of Kentucky College of Medicine, Lexington, Kentucky, US
[6]Faculty of Education, The University of Hong Kong, Hong Kong, PRC

ABSTRACT

A quasi-experimental study with an experimental group (N=195) and a control group (N=71) was conducted to examine the effectiveness of a leadership and intrapersonal development subject at The Hong Kong Polytechnic University. Results showed that there were no significant differences between the two groups in terms of gender ratio, age, and background family characteristics. Analyses using analyses of covariance controlling for pretest differences between the two groups revealed that students in the experimental

[*] Correspondence: Professor Daniel TL Shek, PhD, FHKPS, BBS, JP, Chair Professor of Applied Social Sciences, Faculty of Health and Social Sciences, Department of Applied Social Sciences, The Hong Kong Polytechnic University, Room HJ407, Core H, Hunghom, Hong Kong.. E-mail: daniel.shek@polyu.edu.hk

group generally showed higher levels in psychosocial competence in terms of a composite variable including resilience, social competence, emotional competence, cognitive competence, behavioral competence, self-determination, self-efficacy, and beliefs in the future. In conjunction with other sources of evaluation findings, the present study suggests that this subject is able to promote the holistic development of Chinese university students in Hong Kong.

INTRODUCTION

How can we know whether an intervention is effective or not? One answer to this question is to examine changes in the program participants after they have joined the program. A common strategy to assess changes in program participants is to ask the participants via subjective outcome evaluation or the client satisfaction approach. While the subjective outcome evaluation approach is widely used and easily done, it is also widely criticized as not scientific. Instead of focusing on the effectiveness of the program, subjective outcome may only assess whether the program participants are "happy" or not (1-2).

In the mainstream evaluation literature particularly in the medical sciences (e.g., pediatrics and psychiatry), objective outcome evaluation using experimental designs is still regarded as the "gold standard" for assessing program effectiveness. The prime purpose of an experiment is to assess whether an intervention (independent variable) affects the outcomes (dependent variables) with the minimal confounding effects of irrelevant factors (extraneous variables). In service settings without much resource, a typical approach is to collect pretest and posttest data based on the objective measures and evaluate whether the participants have improved after joining the program (3-5). For example, in a course that attempts to promote creativity in the students, pretest and posttest data based on a standardized creativity test are collected from the participants. If posttest creativity scores are higher than pretest creativity scores, it is usually inferred that the course is effective in promoting creativity in the program participants.

A one-group pretest-posttest design is commonly used to assess the effectiveness of an intervention. Brannick, Miles and Kisamore (6) examined the correlation between mastery and self-efficacy in university students. Students taking a course on research methods in psychology were invited to respond to measures of mastery and self-efficacy at the beginning and at the end of the subject. Results showed that perceived self-efficacy improved after taking the course and the authors concluded that content mastery, self-efficacy, and calibration were facilitated by instructions. Joiner and Jones (7) investigated the impact of medium of communication on the cognitive skills of the students. Based on the responses of 73 students at pretest and posttest under two conditions, students' quality of arguments was examined. Results showed that there were no statistcially significant differences between pretest and posttest scores. Suwantarathip and Wichadee (8) studied the impacts of cooperative learning on anxiety and proficiency in an English class using cooperative learning strategy. Standardized Foreign Language Classroom Anxiety Scale and two proficiency tests covering reading and writing skills were used as the outcome measures. Results showed that language anxiety decreased and language proficiency increased over time. The students also showed favorable attitude to cooperative learning strategy.

While evaluation based on a one group pretest-posttest design is easily carried out in practice settings, there are two limitations. First, the usefulness of this approach depends on whether we have valid and reliable objective outcome variables. Actually, without validated objective outcome measures, it is difficult to objectively assess program outcomes. Second, there are alternative explanations for the change in behavior assessed by the objective outcome measures (i.e., threats to internal validity). There are several threats to internal validity in a design in which pretest and posttest data are collected from the intervention group only.

Primarily, time-related factors may constitute threats to the internal validity of a pretest-posttest design. First, historical events taking place between pretest and posttest may affect the posttest score. One example is that in a treatment group for depression, reduction in depressive symptoms at posttest may simply be due to improvement in the economy. Second, test reactivity may affect the posttest. For example, if the pretest experience is no good, this experience would affect the posttest scores in a pretest-posttest design. The third time threat is maturation where it is argued that posttest change is a reflection of the normal maturation of the participants. Fourth, instrumentation is another time threat to be considered. For example, the psychometric properties of a measure of civic responsibility may be substantially impaired by some recent incidents about responsibility problems of adolescents. Finally, regression to the mean is another time threat. For example, if the pretest scores fall within the lower end of a distribution, improvement of posttest score may simply be a statistical artifact owing to systematic increase in the scores over time.

One useful strategy that can be used to deal with time threat is to include a control group in the study. Nevertheless, even if the inclusion of a control group, it is noteworthy that there is still the possibility of "group" threat. In other words, differences between the experimental group and control group may be due to pre-existing group differences (9-10).

At The Hong Kong Polytechnic University, all students admitted under the New Undergraduate Curriculum will be required to take a course to fulfill the requirement in the area on Leadership and Intrapersonal Development starting from 2012/13 academic year. A subject entitled "Tomorrow's Leaders" has been developed by the first author to fulfill this requirement. Utilizing the literature on positive youth development constructs, including self-understanding, resilience, cognitive competence, social competence, emotional competence, moral competence, integrity, spirituality, and clear and positive identity, students are helped to enhance their self-understanding and interpersonal relationship. To test out the curriculum, "Tomorrow's Leaders" was offered in the second term of 2010/11 academic year on a pilot basis and different evaluation strategies were used to evaluate the subject. Generally speaking, evaluation based on different strategies showed that the subject was able to promote the psychosocial competence of the students (11-17).

While evaluation findings based on the first piloting exercise are very encouraging, there are two limitations involved. First, there is a need to replicate the findings to rule out the possibility that the favorable findings are based on sheer chance effect. Second, as far as objective outcome evaluation is concerned, only a one-group pretest-posttest design was used. As mentioned above, a one-group pretest-posttest design is a necessary but not sufficient condition for establishing the claim that an intervention leads to positive changes in the program participants. By adding a control group, most of the time threats can be removed.

OUR STUDY

The course titled "Tomorrow's Leaders" was piloted for the second time in the first term of 2011/12 school year in The Hong Kong Polytechnic University. The subjects of the Experimental Group were recruited from four classes attending the course (N = 195). The subjects for the Control Group (N =71) were recruited from three classes of students attending other courses, including "Self Service and Community", "Contemporary Chinese Society and Popular Culture", and "Global China".

During the first lecture, a questionnaire containing items on holistic youth development was distributed to the students in the Experimental Group and Control Group to complete the pretest assessment. The students were invited to participate in the study in a voluntary manner and informed consent was obtained. They were instructed to complete the questionnaire after class and returned the questionnaire in the next lecture. To match the pretest data with the posttest data, informants were asked to put down their date of birth (month and date) and the last four digits of their Hong Kong Identity Card numbers.

At Lecture 13, the same questionnaire was distributed to students in the Experimental Group and Control Group who had completed the questionnaire at the pretest. Again, they were instructed to complete the questionnaire after class and returned the questionnaire in the next lecture.

Instruments

At both the pretest and posttest, the participants were invited to respond to a questionnaire including measures of positive youth development, thriving, life satisfaction, adolescent problem behavior, and demographic information. In this chapter, findings based on the Chinese Positive Youth Development Scale (CPYDS) are reported.

The CPYDS was developed to assess holistic development in the program participants and it was found to possess adequate psychometric properties (18). Based on reliability analyses of both the pretest and posttest data in the present study, some slight modifications in the composition of the 13 subscales of the CPYDS are shown as follows:

1. Resilience Subscale (6 items)
2. Social Competence Subscale (7 items)
3. Emotional Competence Subscale (6 items)
4. Cognitive Competence Subscale (6 items)
5. Behavioral Competence Subscale (modified 5 items)
6. Moral Competence Subscale (6 items)
7. Self-Determination Subscale (modified 5 items)
8. Self-Efficacy Subscale (modified 2 items)
9. Beliefs in the Future Subscale (modified 3 items)
10. Clear and Positive Identity Subscale (7 items)
11. Spirituality Subscale (7 items)
12. Bonding Subscale (6 items)
13. Prosocial Norms Subscale (5 items)

Several composite indices based on the above measures were formed in the analyses. As the course did not focus on bonding and prosocial norms, a composite score based on 11 subscales (i.e., resilience, emotional competence, social competence, cognitive competence, behavioral competence, moral competence, self-determination, self-efficacy, beliefs in the future, clear and positive identity, and spirituality) was formed. Besides, a composite measure based on 8 measures of psychosocial competence (i.e., resilience, emotional competence, social competence, cognitive competence, behavioral competence, self-determination, self-efficacy, and beliefs in the future) was used. Finally, higher-order factors based on cognitive-behavioral competence and positive identity (19) were examined.

FINDINGS

Concerning the reliability of the measures covered in this chapter, analyses showed that the measures were basically internally consistent. The findings are presented in Table 1. To examine whether there were intrinsic differences between the Experimental Group and Control Group, results showed that the two groups did not differ in terms of gender ratio, age, family size, parental marital status, perceived family happiness, and perceived school adjustment.

To control for the possible influence of pretest scores, analyses of covariance controlling for pretest differences between the Experimental Group and Control Group were carried out. Using the composite variable based on 11 subscales, ANCOVA analyses showed that the two groups did not differ in the posttest scores (Table 2). However, separate analyses of pretest and posttest differences showed that while the improvement in the Experimental Group was significant, the related change in the Control Group was not significant (Table 3).

Table 1. Coefficient alphas and mean inter-item correlation coefficients of different measures at pretest and posttest

Variables	Pretest	Posttest
CPYDS (11 domains)	.95 (.22)	.96 (.25)
CBC (Higher order factor)	.85 (.26)	.86 (.29)
PIT (Higher order factor)	.86 (.32)	.87 (.33)
CPYDS (8 domains)	.93 (.23)	.94 (.26)
Resilience	.80 (.40)	.83 (.50)
Social Competence	.82 (.40)	.81 (.38)
Cognitive Competence	.76 (.35)	.80 (.41)
Emotional Competence	.76 (.35)	.80 (.40)
Behavioral Competence	.61 (.23)	.61 (.25)
Self-Determination	.78 (.42)	.76 (.39)
Self-Efficacy	.83 (.38)	.85 (.41)
Beliefs in the Future	.84 (.43)	.84 (.42)
Spirituality	.82 (.43)	.87 (.54)
Clear and Positive Identity	.81 (.38)	.82 (.40)
Moral Competence	.72 (.30)	.75 (.33)

- CPYDS [Chinese Positive Youth Development Scale] (11 domains): mean of resilience, emotional competence, social competence, cognitive competence, behavioral competence, moral competence, self-determination, self-efficacy, beliefs in the future, clear and positive identity, and spirituality.
- CPYDS (8 domains): mean of resilience, emotional competence, social competence, cognitive competence, behavioral competence, self-determination, self-efficacy, and beliefs in the future.
- CBC [Cognitive-behavioral Competence]: mean of self-determination, behavioral competence, and cognitive competence
- PIT [Positive Identity]: mean of beliefs in the future and clear and positive identity

Table 2. Differences between Experimental Group and Control Group in terms of post-test scores after controlling for pretest differences

Variables	Experimental	Control	F value	E > C
Composite Variable				
CPYDS (11 domains)	4.67	4.62	1.03	Y
CBC (Higher order factor)	4.70	4.53	9.87**	Y
PIT (Higher order factor)	4.56	4.51	0.72	Y
CPYDS (8 domains)	4.62	4.53	3.23[a]	Y
Individual Subscale Variable				
Resilience	4.97	4.89	1.07	Y
Social Competence	4.79	4.75	0.52	Y
Cognitive Competence	4.69	4.53	5.54*	Y
Emotional Competence	4.47	4.43	0.27	Y
Behavioral Competence	4.59	4.48	2.23	Y
Self-Determination	4.83	4.61	9.19**	Y
Self-Efficacy	4.00	3.76	4.92*	Y
Beliefs in the Future	4.69	4.53	3.18[a]	Y
Individual Item Variable				
Item a (resilience)	5.00	4.76	4.46*	Y
Item b (resilience)	5.01	4.74	2.93[a]	Y
Item c (self-understanding)	4.64	4.41	3.38[a]	Y
Item d (coping)	4.81	4.61	2.91*	Y
Item e (spiritual value)	5.13	4.67	4.00*	Y
Item f (fullness of life)	5.37	4.92	2.86[a]	Y

**$p < .01$; *$p < .05$; a $p < .05$ (one-tailed).

- CPYDS (11 domains): mean of resilience, emotional competence, social competence, cognitive competence, behavioral competence, moral competence, self-determination, self-efficacy, beliefs in the future, clear and positive identity, and spirituality.
- CPYDS (8 domains): mean of resilience, emotional competence, social competence, cognitive competence, behavioral competence, self-determination, self-efficacy, and beliefs in the future.
- *Item a*: My belief is that even if tomorrow will become worse, I will still live in a good manner. (Resilience Subscale)
- *Item b*: I believe problems in life can be resolved. (Resilience Subscale)

- *Item c*: I know my strengths and weaknesses. (Clear and Positive Identity Subscale)
- *Item d*: I am able to handle difficulties and challenges in my life. (Thriving Scale)
- *Item e*: I believe that spiritual riches are more important than material prosperity. (Thriving Scale)
- *Item f*: My life is colorful and full of excitements. (Spirituality Subscale)

Table 3. Pretest and posttest differences in the Experimental Group and Control Group in terms of composite variables

Variable	Group	Pretest Score	Posttest Mean	t-value
CPYDS (11 domains)	Experimental	4.624	4.713	-3.74***
	Control	4.449	4.522	-1.44ns
Cognitive-behavioral competence (higher-order factor)	Experimental	4.559	4.715	-5.10***
	Control	4.492	4.504	-0.21ns
Positive Identity factor (higher-order factor)	Experimental	4.596	4.623	-0.76ns
	Control	4.339	4.380	-0.76ns
CPYDS (8 domains)	Experimental	4.553	4.654	-3.88***
	Control	4.409	4.455	-0.84ns

*** $p < .001$; ns = non-significant.

Further analyses based on the higher-order factors of the Chinese Positive Youth Development Scale revealed that the Experimental Group showed higher posttest cognitive-behavioral competence than did the Control Group (see Table 1). Again, separate analyses of pretest and posttest differences showed that while the improvement in the Experimental Group was significant, no significant change could be found in the Control Group (Table 3).

As the findings showed that there were significant differences between the two groups in terms of cognitive-behavioral competence, another composite score based on eight cognitive-behavioral measures was created. Analyses showed that there was significant difference between these two groups at the posttest. Again, while the posttest score was significantly higher in the Experimental Group, there was no difference between the pre- post-test scores in the Control Group. Analyses based on subscales showed that the two groups differed in terms of posttest scores in the domains of cognitive competence, self-determination, and self-efficacy (see Table 1). Although there were non-significant differences on some subscales, analyses using Sign Test showed that the mean of the Experimental Group was consistently higher than those of the Control Group on all eight subscales ($p < .05$). Furthermore, results showed that the two groups differed on some items, with some examples shown in Table 1.

DISCUSSION

Course evaluation has been regarded as an important task in the context of higher education, with subjective outcome evaluation as the most common form of evaluation. In fact, a review of the literature shows that many validated measures have been developed in the West. For example, Spooren, Mortelmans and Denekens (20) developed a conceptual framework on teaching quality with 8 domains and 22 sub-domains. The major dimensions were course objectives, subject matter, course structure, teaching activities, course materials, course feasibility, coaching, and evaluation. Utilizing confirmatory factor analyses, 10 final empirically supported dimensions were found, including clarity of objectives, value of subject matter, build-up of subject matter, presentation skills, harmony organization course – learning process, contribution to understanding the subject, course difficulty, help of the teacher during the learning process, authenticity of examination(s) and formative examination(s). In the Teacher Effectiveness Survey (21), five dimensions including teaching quality, feedback and support, learning, workload, and overall evaluation were identified. In the Course Experience Questionnaire, Waugh (22) identified six dimensions, including student support, learning resources, learning community, intellectual motivation, course organization, and graduate qualities. Finally, Kim, Damewood and Hodge (23) proposed eight broad dimensions underlying course evaluation, including teacher character traits, management of the class, assignments, course design, testing, grading, feedback, and course materials.

While subjective outcome evaluation is a convenient approach, it is not designed to examine the effect of an intervention on students. That is, subjective outcome evaluation cannot establish the influence of an intervention (i.e., a course) on the outcomes of the students. Alternatively, there are views arguing that adoption of an experimental approach is a superior form of evaluation. In the context of human services, quasi-experimental approach (i.e., use of an experimental group and a control group without random assignment of subjects to each group) is a recommended approach in program evaluation. For example, adopting a quasi-experimental approach, St. Pierre and her associates (24) examined the effectiveness of the SMART program over time. In Hong Kong, a quasi-experimental study was conducted to examine the effectiveness of the Project ASTRO which attempted to prevent substance abuse in young people (25).

The objective outcome evaluation findings reported in this chapter are generally positive and they are consistent with the original expectations. Although there was no difference between the two groups in terms of the CPYDS (11 domains) variable, posttest scores were significantly higher than pretest scores in the Experimental Group but not in the Control Group. Results also showed that the Experimental Group performed better than did the Control Group based on the CPYDS (8 domains) composite variable, individual subscales, and individual items levels. The program effect could be regarded as encouraging in view of the short duration of the intervention program which lasted for about 14 weeks. It is noteworthy that this is the first known scientific study which examined the effectiveness of a credit-bearing course aiming at promoting psychosocial competencies in university students in different Chinese communities. As Shek and Yu (26) pointed out, validated adolescent prevention and positive youth development programs in Asia are sparse. Hence, the present study is a groundbreaking contribution to the existing literature.

Research findings suggest that there are developmental issues amongst university students that deserve our attention, such as mental health problems, narcissism, political apathy, and ethical issues. At the same time, there are views suggesting that contemporary university education fails to promote holistic development in university students. In view of these phenomena, it is (27,28) argued that there is a need to design credit-bearing courses on positive youth development to promote holistic development in university students. The present finding suggests that a credit-bearing course is a promising approach to promote psychosocial competence in university students. Furthermore, this approach is consistent with the public health principle of universal prevention.

The present findings are consistent with the evaluation findings based on other evaluation strategies in both the first and second piloting exercises. First, post-course subjective outcome evaluation findings in both piloting exercises showed that students generally had positive perceptions of the subject and teacher, and the subject was perceived as helpful to them in the domains of intrapersonal development and leadership. Second, post-lecture subjective outcome evaluation showed that the students generally had positive perception of the lecture content and the lecture process. Third, process evaluation in both exercises consistently showed that program adherence was high and the subject implementation process was good. Fourth, qualitative studies based on student reflections and focus groups also consistently showed that the students had positive perceptions of the subject, teacher, and benefits gained from taking this subject. In short, an integration of evaluation findings based on these two piloting exercises provides support for the claim that "Tomorrow's Leaders" can promote psychosocial competencies in university students in Hong Kong.

However, there are three points that should be noted when the present findings are interpreted. First, as a cross sectional design was used, there is a need to examine the long-term effectiveness of the subject via the use of longitudinal research designs. In particular, it is necessary to examine the real-life relevance of the materials learned from the subject. One possible evaluation strategy is to ask students to write personal reflections after taking this course. This strategy has proven to be very effective in the Project P.A.T.H.S. in Hong Kong (29-33). Besides, the use of the repertory grid technique would be a useful strategy to examine the perceived change in the program participants (34).

Second, although the addition of a control group can strengthen the internal validity of the study, there are still threats to the internal validity of the study. For example, intrinsic differences between the groups may be a possible confounding factor inflating the differences between the two groups. Hence, random selection and random assignment of subjects to the experimental and control conditions would be helpful to further uncover the effectiveness of the subject.

Finally, besides the indicators based on the Chinese Positive Youth Development Scale (CPYDS), other indicators reflecting adolescent developmental issues such as narcissism, empathy, and civic engagement should be developed and used in future studies. Despite these limitations, the present study is a constructive response to those views suggesting that contemporary university education cannot promote holistic development of university students (35-39).

ACKNOWLEDGMENTS

This work and the course on "Tomorrow's Leaders" are financially supported by The Hong Kong Polytechnic University. Members of the Curriculum Development Team include Daniel T.L. Shek, Yat Hung Chui, Siu Wai Lit, Yida Y.H. Chung, Sowa Ngai, Yammy L.Y. Chak, Pik Fong Tsui, Cecilia M.S. Ma, Lu Yu and Moon Y.M. Law. This chapter has been published as a paper in the International Journal on Disability and Human Development, 2013;12(2). Permission has been obtained from De Gruyter to re-publish in this modified form.

REFERENCES

[1] LaSala MC. Client satisfaction: consideration of correlates and response bias. Fam Soc 1997;78:54-64.

[2] Lebow JL. Research assessing consumer satisfaction with mental health treatment: a review of findings. Eval Program Plann 1983;6:211-36.

[3] Thyer B. Evaluation of social work practice in the new millennium: myths and realities. In: Shek DTL, Lam MC, Au CF, Lee JJ, editors. Entering a new millennium: advances in social welfare service and research. Hong Kong: New Asia College and the Chinese University Press, The Chinese University of Hong Kong, 2002:3–18.

[4] Rubin A, Babbie E. Research methods for social work. Delmont, CA: Thomson Learning, 2008.

[5] Singleton RA, Straits BC. Approaches to social research. New York: Oxford University Press, 2005.

[6] Brannick MT, Miles DE, Kisamore JL. Calibration between student mastery and self-efficacy. Stud High Educ 2005;30:473-83.

[7] Joiner R, Jones S. The effects of communication medium on argumentation and the development of critical thinking. Int J Educ Res 2003;39:861-71.

[8] Suwantarathip O, Wichadee S. The impacts of cooperative learning on anxiety and proficiency in an EFL class. Journal of College Teaching & Learning 2010;7:51-7.

[9] Gliner JA, Morgan GA. Research methods in applied settings: an integrated approach to design and analysis. Mahwah, NJ: Erlbaum, 2000.

[10] Gomm R, Needham G, Bullman A. Evaluating research in health and social care. London: Sage, 2000.

[11] Shek DTL, Sun RCF. Promoting psychosocial competencies in university students: evaluation based on a one group pretest-posttest design. Int J Disabil Hum Dev 2012;11:229-34.

[12] Shek DTL, Sun RCF. Promoting leadership and intrapersonal competence in university students: what can we learn from Hong Kong? Int J Disabil Hum Dev 2012;11:221-8.

[13] Shek DTL, Sun RCF. Process evaluation of a positive youth development course in a university setting in Hong Kong. Int J Disabil Hum Dev 2012;11:235-41.

[14] Shek DTL, Sun RCF. Qualitative evaluation of a positive youth development course in a university setting in Hong Kong. Int J Disabil Hum Dev 2012;11:243-8.

[15] Shek DTL, Sun RCF. Focus group evaluation of a positive youth development course in a university in Hong Kong. Int J Disabil Hum Dev 2012;11:249-54.

[16] Shek DTL, Sun RCF, Chui YH, Lit SW, Yuen WWW, Chung YYH, Ngai SW. Development and evaluation of a positive youth development course for university students in Hong Kong. ScientificWorldJournal 2012; Article ID 263731, 8 pages. DOI: 10.1100/2012/263731.

[17] Shek DTL. Post-lecture evaluation of a positive youth development subject for university students in Hong Kong. ScientificWorldJournal 2012, Article ID 934679, 8 pages. DOI: 10.1100/2012/934679.

[18] Shek DTL, Siu AMH, Lee TY. The Chinese Positive Youth development Scale: a validation study. Res Soc Work Pract 2007;17:380–91.

[19] Shek DTL, Ma CMS. Dimensionality of the Chinese Positive Youth Development Scale: confirmatory factor analyses. Soc Indic Res 2010;98:41–59.

[20] Spooren P, Mortelmans D, Denekens J. Student evaluation of teaching quality in higher education: development of an instrument based on 10 Likert-scales. Assessment and Evaluation in Higher Education 2007;32:667-79.

[21] Stringer M, Irwing P. Students' evaluations of teaching effectiveness: a structural modeling approach. Brit J Educ Psychol 1998;68:409-26.

[22] Waugh RF. The course experience questionnaire: a Rasch measurement model analysis. Higher Education Research and Development 1998;17:45-64.

[23] Kim C, Damewood E, Hodge N. Professor attitude: its effect on teaching evaluations. Journal of Management Education 2000;24:458-73.

[24] St Pierre TL, Kaltreider DL, Mark MM, Aikin KJ. Drug prevention in a community setting: a longitudinal study of the relative effectiveness of a three-year primary prevention program in Boys and Girls Clubs across the nation. Am J Com Psychol 1992;20:673-706.

[25] Lam CW, Shek DTL. Objective outcome evaluation of a drug prevention program for high-risk youths in Hong Kong: the Project Astro. Int J Child Health Hum Dev 2011;4:361-76.

[26] Shek DTL, Yu L. A review of validated youth prevention and positive youth development programs in Asia. Int J Adolesc Med Health 2011;23:317-24.
[27] Shek DTL. Nurturing holistic development of university students in Hong Kong: where are we and where should we go? ScientificWorldJournal 2010;10:563-75.
[28] Shek DTL, Wong KK. Do adolescent developmental issues disappear overnight? Reflections about holistic development in university students. ScientificWorldJournal 2011;11:353-61.
[29] Shek DTL, Ma CMS, Tang CYP. Predictors of subjective outcome evaluation findings in a positive youth development program in Hong Kong. Int J Disabil Hum Dev 2011;10:249-55.
[30] Shek DTL, Sun RCF, Merrick J. Training programs and implementation process of positive youth development programs. Int J Adolesc Med Health 2011;23:303-4.
[31] Shek DTL, Ma HK, Sun RCF. A brief overview of adolescent developmental problems in Hong Kong. ScientificWorldJournal 2011;11:2243-56.
[32] Shek DTL, Ma HK, Sun RCF. Development of a new curriculum in a positive youth development program: the Project P.A.T.H.S. in Hong Kong. ScientificWorldJournal 2011;11:2207-18.
[33] Shek DTL. Quality of life research: responses to emerging issues in a changing world. Soc Indic Res 2011;100:371-4.
[34] Shek DTL. Evaluation of a positive youth development program based on the repertory grid test. ScientificWorldJournal 2012, Article ID 372752, 12 pages. DOI: 10.1100/2012/372752.
[35] Bok D. Our underachieving colleges: a candid look at how much students learn and why they should be learning more. Princeton: Princeton University Press, 2006.
[36] Lewis HR. Excellence without a soul: how a great university forgot education. New York: Public Affairs Publishing, 2006.
[37] Tull A. What they're reading - excellence without a soul: how a great university forgot education. J Coll Character 2007;8:1–2.
[38] Dalton J, Crosby P. The neglected inner lives of college students. J Coll Character 2006;7:1–2.
[39] Dalton J, Crosby P. Being and having: shouldn't excellence in higher education (and people) be a measure of what one does rather than what one has? J Coll Character 2007;9:1–5.

ACKNOWLEDGEMENTS

In: Chinese Adolescent Development ISBN: 978-1-62618-622-4
Editors: Daniel TL Shek, Rachel CF Sun, Joav Merrick © 2013 Nova Science Publishers, Inc.

Chapter 13

About the Editors

Daniel TL Shek, PhD, FHKPS, BBS, JP, is Chair Professor of Applied Social Sciences, Department of Applied Social Sciences, Hong Kong Polytechnic University, Hunghom, Hong Kong, PRC, Advisory Professor of East China Normal University and Honorary Professor of Kiang Wu Nursing College of Macau. He is Chief Editor of *Journal of Youth Studies*, Consulting Editor of *Journal of Clinical Psychology*, international consultant of *American Journal of Family Therapy*, and editorial board member of *Social Indicators Research, International Journal of Adolescent Medicine and Health, The Scientific World Journal (Child Health and Human Development and Holistic Health and Medicine domains), Asian Journal of Counseling, International Journal of Disability and Human Development,* and *Bentham Open Family Studies Journal*. He has served in many government advisory bodies, including the Action Committee against Narcotics, Commission on Youth, Fight Crime Committee and Family Council. He has published numerous books, book chapters and more than 300 scientific articles in international refereed journals. E-mail: daniel.shek@polyu.edu.hk

Rachel CF Sun, PhD, is assistant professor at the Faculty of Education, The University of Hong Kong, Hong Kong, PRC. She teaches in the areas of psychology of teaching and learning, and child and adolescent development. Her research areas include academic achievement motivation, student misbehavior, school satisfaction, life satisfaction, positive youth development, adolescent suicidal ideation and psychological health. She is a co-principal investigator of a huge and pioneering positive youth development project in Hong Kong. She is an Executive Committee member of the Society of Boys' Centres, and a member of the Editorial Board of *Research on Social Work Practice.* E-mail: rachels@hku.hk

Joav Merrick, MD, MMedSci, DMSc, is professor of pediatrics, child health and human development affiliated with Kentucky Children's Hospital, University of Kentucky, Lexington, United States and the Division of Pediatrics, Hadassah Hebrew University Medical Centers, Mt Scopus Campus, Jerusalem, Israel, the medical director of the Health Services, Division for Intellectual and Developmental Disabilities, Ministry of Social Affairs and Social Services, Jerusalem, the founder and director of the National Institute of Child Health and Human Development in Israel. Numerous publications in the field of pediatrics, child health and human development, rehabilitation, intellectual disability, disability, health, welfare, abuse, advocacy, quality of life and prevention. Received the Peter Sabroe Child Award for outstanding work on behalf of Danish Children in 1985 and the International LEGO-Prize ("The Children's Nobel Prize") for an extraordinary contribution towards improvement in child welfare and well-being in 1987. E-mail: jmerrick@zahav.net.il

In: Chinese Adolescent Development ISBN: 978-1-62618-622-4
Editors: Daniel TL Shek, Rachel CF Sun, Joav Merrick © 2013 Nova Science Publishers, Inc.

Chapter 14

About the Department of Applied Social Sciences, the Hong Kong Polytechnic University

The Department of Applied Social Sciences (APSS) of The Hong Kong Polytechnic University is one of the largest and most vibrant centres in the region dedicated to the education and training of professional social workers, social policy and welfare administrators, psychologists and counselors in Hong Kong.

The Department started as the Institute of Social Work Training in 1973. It joined the Hong Kong Polytechnic in 1977 and became its School of Social Work. The School was eventually renamed the Department of Applied Social Sciences. APSS celebrated its 35th anniversary in the academic year of 2007/08. Currently there are 93 full-time academics, over 80 research/project staff, 20 fieldwork supervisors and 34 colleagues in other categories, including administrative and supporting personnel.

The Department has six thriving Research Centres: Centre for Social Policy Studies, China Research and Development Network, Network for Health and Welfare Studies, Professional Practice and Assessment Centre, Centre for Third Sector Studies, and the Manulife Centre for Children with Specific Learning Disabilities, providing platforms for collaborative research and practice projects with government departments and NGOs.

The Department of Applied Social Sciences offers taught programs in the fields of Social Work, Social Policy and Administration, Counseling, and Applied Psychology, as well as research degrees at MPhil and PhD levels. In 2008/09, APSS offered some 20 Programs for Higher Diploma, Degree, Postgraduate, MPhil and PhD students. There are currently about 1,500 students enrolled in the various APSS programs and we have graduated more than 14,000 students over the years.

In the past decade, the Department has successfully expanded into the Chinese mainland. The Department currently offers a MSW(China) Program in collaboration with Peking University and a Joint PolyU-PekingU Social Work Research Centre has been established to foster research in social work and social policy.

Contact

Professor Daniel TL Shek, PhD, FHKPS, BBS, JP
Chair Professor of Applied Social Sciences
Department of Applied Social Sciences
The Hong Kong Polytechnic University
Hunghom, Hong Kong
E-mail: daniel.shek@polyu.edu.hk

In: Chinese Adolescent Development ISBN: 978-1-62618-622-4
Editors: Daniel TL Shek, Rachel CF Sun, Joav Merrick © 2013 Nova Science Publishers, Inc.

Chapter 15

About the National Institute of Child Health and Human Development in Israel

The National Institute of Child Health and Human Development (NICHD) in Israel was established in 1998 as a virtual institute under the auspices of the Medical Director, Ministry of Social Affairs and Social Services in order to function as the research arm for the Office of the Medical Director. In 1998 the National Council for Child Health and Pediatrics, Ministry of Health and in 1999 the Director General and Deputy Director General of the Ministry of Health endorsed the establishment of the NICHD. In 2011 the NICHD became affiliated with the Division of Pediatrics, Hadassah Hebrew University Medical Center, Mt Scopus Campus in Jerusalem.

Mission

The mission of a National Institute for Child Health and Human Development in Israel is to provide an academic focal point for the scholarly interdisciplinary study of child life, health, public health, welfare, disability, rehabilitation, intellectual disability and related aspects of human development. This mission includes research, teaching, clinical work, information and public service activities in the field of child health and human development.

Service and Academic Activities

Over the years many activities became focused in the south of Israel due to collaboration with various professionals at the Faculty of Health Sciences (FOHS) at the Ben Gurion University of the Negev (BGU). Since 2000 an affiliation with the Zusman Child Development Center at the Pediatric Division of Soroka University Medical Center has resulted in collaboration around the establishment of the Down Syndrome Clinic at that center. In 2002 a full course on "Disability" was established at the Recanati School for Allied Professions in the Community, FOHS, BGU and in 2005 collaboration was started with the Primary Care Unit of the faculty and disability became part of the master of public health course on "Children and society". In the academic year 2005-2006 a one semester course on "Aging with disability" was started as part of the master of science program in gerontology in our collaboration with the Center for Multidisciplinary Research in Aging. In 2010 collaborations with the Division of Pediatrics, Hadassah Hebrew University Medical Center, Jerusalem, Israel around the National Down Syndrome Center and teaching students and residents about intellectual and developmental disabilities as part of their training at this campus.

RESEARCH ACTIVITIES

The affiliated staff have over the years published work from projects and research activities in this national and international collaboration. In the year 2000 the International Journal of Adolescent Medicine and Health and in 2005 the International Journal on Disability and Human Development of De Gruyter Publishing House (Berlin and New York) were affiliated with the National Institute of Child Health and Human Development. From 2008 also the International Journal of Child Health and Human Development (Nova Science, New York), the International Journal of Child and Adolescent Health (Nova Science) and the Journal of Pain Management (Nova Science) affiliated and from 2009 the International Public Health Journal (Nova Science) and Journal of Alternative Medicine Research (Nova Science). All peer-reviewed international journals.

NATIONAL COLLABORATIONS

Nationally the NICHD works in collaboration with the Faculty of Health Sciences, Ben Gurion University of the Negev; Department of Physical Therapy, Sackler School of Medicine, Tel Aviv University; Autism Center, Assaf HaRofeh Medical Center; National Rett and PKU Centers at Chaim Sheba Medical Center, Tel HaShomer; Department of Physiotherapy, Haifa University; Department of Education, Bar Ilan University, Ramat Gan, Faculty of Social Sciences and Health Sciences; College of Judea and Samaria in Ariel and in 2011 affiliation with Center for Pediatric Chronic Diseases and National Center for Down Syndrome, Department of Pediatrics, Hadassah Hebrew University Medical Center, Mount Scopus Campus, Jerusalem.

INTERNATIONAL COLLABORATIONS

Internationally with the Department of Disability and Human Development, College of Applied Health Sciences, University of Illinois at Chicago; Strong Center for Developmental Disabilities, Golisano Children's Hospital at Strong, University of Rochester School of Medicine and Dentistry, New York; Centre on Intellectual Disabilities, University of Albany, New York; Centre for Chronic Disease Prevention and Control, Health Canada, Ottawa; Chandler Medical Center and Children's Hospital, Kentucky Children's Hospital, Section of Adolescent Medicine, University of Kentucky, Lexington; Chronic Disease Prevention and Control Research Center, Baylor College of Medicine, Houston, Texas; Division of Neuroscience, Department of Psychiatry, Columbia University, New York; Institute for the

Study of Disadvantage and Disability, Atlanta; Center for Autism and Related Disorders, Department Psychiatry, Children's Hospital Boston, Boston; Department of Paediatrics, Child Health and Adolescent Medicine, Children's Hospital at Westmead, Westmead, Australia; International Centre for the Study of Occupational and Mental Health, Düsseldorf, Germany; Centre for Advanced Studies in Nursing, Department of General Practice and Primary Care, University of Aberdeen, Aberdeen, United Kingdom; Quality of Life Research Center, Copenhagen, Denmark; Nordic School of Public Health, Gottenburg, Sweden, Scandinavian Institute of Quality of Working Life, Oslo, Norway; The Department of Applied Social Sciences (APSS) of The Hong Kong Polytechnic University Hong Kong.

TARGETS

Our focus is on research, international collaborations, clinical work, teaching and policy in health, disability and human development and to establish the NICHD as a permanent institute at one of the residential care centers for persons with intellectual disability in Israel in order to conduct model research and together with the four university schools of public health/medicine in Israel establish a national master and doctoral program in disability and human development at the institute to secure the next generation of professionals working in this often non-prestigious/low-status field of work.

Contact

Joav Merrick, MD, DMSc
Professor of Pediatrics, Child Health and Human Development
Medical Director, Health Services, Division for Intellectual and Developmental Disabilities, Ministry of Social Affairs and Social Services, POB 1260, IL-91012 Jerusalem, Israel.
E-mail: jmerrick@zahav.net.il

In: Chinese Adolescent Development ISBN: 978-1-62618-622-4
Editors: Daniel TL Shek, Rachel CF Sun, Joav Merrick © 2013 Nova Science Publishers, Inc.

Chapter 16

ABOUT THE BOOK SERIES "PEDIATRICS, CHILD AND ADOLESCENT HEALTH"

Pediatrics, child and adolescent health is a book series with publications from a multidisciplinary group of researchers, practitioners and clinicians for an international professional forum interested in the broad spectrum of pediatric medicine, child health, adolescent health and human development.

- Merrick J, ed. Child and adolescent health yearbook 2011. New York: Nova Science, 2012.
- Merrick J, ed. Child and adolescent health yearbook 2012. New York: Nova Science, 2012.
- Roach RR, Greydanus DE, Patel DR, Homnick DN, Merrick J, eds. Tropical pediatrics: A public health concern of international proportions. New York: Nova Science, 2012.
- Merrick J, ed. Child health and human development yearbook 2011. New York: Nova Science, 2012.
- Merrick J, ed. Child health and human development yearbook 2012. New York: Nova Science, 2012.
- Shek DTL, Sun RCF, Merrick J, eds. Developmental issues in Chinese adolescents. New York: Nova Science, 2012.
- Shek DTL, Sun RCF, Merrick J, eds. Positive youth development: Theory, research and application. New York: Nova Science, 2012.
- Zachor DA, Merrick J, eds. Understanding autism spectrum disorder: Current research aspects. New York: Nova Science, 2012.
- Ma HK, Shek DTL, Merrick J, eds. Positive youth development: A new school curriculum to tackle adolescent developmental issues. New York: Nova Science, 2012.
- Wood D, Reiss JG, Ferris ME, Edwards LR, Merrick J, eds. Transition from pediatric to adult medical care. New York: Nova Science, 2012.

Contact

Professor Joav Merrick, MD, MMedSci, DMSc
Medical Director, Medical Services

Division for Intellectual and Developmental Disabilities
Ministry of Social Affairs and Social Services
POBox 1260, IL-91012 Jerusalem, Israel
E-mail: jmerrick@zahav.net.il

INDEX

C

D

E

I

J

K

L

M

N

O

P

Q

R

T

U

V

W

Y